REIKI
for Life

The Complete Guide

to Reiki Practice

for Levels 1, 2 & 3

Penelope Quest

JEREMY P. TARCHER/PENGUIN

a member of Penguin Group (USA) Inc.

New York

JEREMY P. TARCHER/PENGUIN
Published by the Penguin Group
Penguin Group (USA) Inc., 375 Hudson Street, New York, New York 10014, USA •
Penguin Group (Canada), 90 Eglinton Avenue East, Suite 700, Toronto, Ontario M4P 2Y3,
Canada (a division of Pearson Penguin Canada Inc.) • Penguin Books Ltd, 80 Strand,
London WC2R 0RL, England • Penguin Ireland, 25 St Stephen's Green, Dublin 2, Ireland
(a division of Penguin Books Ltd) • Penguin Group (Australia), 250 Camberwell Road,
Camberwell, Victoria 3124, Australia (a division of Pearson Australia Group Pty Ltd) •
Penguin Books India Pvt Ltd, 11 Community Centre, Panchsheel Park, New Delhi–110 017,
India • Penguin Group (NZ), 67 Apollo Drive, Rosedale, North Shore 0632, New Zealand
(a division of Pearson New Zealand Ltd) • Penguin Books (South Africa) (Pty) Ltd,
24 Sturdee Avenue, Rosebank, Johannesburg 2196, South Africa

Penguin Books Ltd, Registered Offices: 80 Strand, London WC2R 0RL, England

Originally published in the UK by Piatkus 2002
First published in the United States by Jeremy P. Tarcher/Penguin 2010
Copyright © 2002, 2009 by Penelope Quest

Most Tarcher/Penguin books are available at special quantity discounts for bulk purchase
for sales promotions, premiums, fund-raising, and educational needs. Special books or book
excerpts also can be created to fit specific needs. For details, write Penguin Group (USA) Inc.
Special Markets, 375 Hudson Street, New York, NY 10014.

Library of Congress Cataloging-in-Publication Data

Quest, Penelope.
Reiki for life: the complete guide to reiki practice for levels 1, 2 & 3 / Penelope Quest.
p.   cm.
ISBN 978-1-58542-790-1
1. Reiki (Healing system)   I. Title.
RZ403.R45Q477   2010   2009051213
615.8'51—dc22

Printed in the United States of America
1 3 5 7 9 10 8 6 4 2

Neither the publisher nor the author is engaged in rendering professional advice or services to the individual reader. The ideas, procedures, and suggestions contained in this book are not intended as a substitute for consulting with your physician. All matters regarding your health require medical supervision.
Neither the author nor the publisher shall be liable or responsible for any loss or damage allegedly arising
from any information or suggestion in this book.

While the author has made every effort to provide accurate telephone numbers and Internet addresses at
the time of publication, neither the publisher nor the author assumes any responsibility for errors, or for
changes that occur after publication. Further, the publisher does not have any control over and does not
assume any responsibility for author or third-party websites or their content.

This book is dedicated to Mikao Usui, without whom the world would not have received the wonderful gift of Reiki.

Acknowledgments

I would like to express my heartfelt gratitude to the many people who have helped, directly or indirectly, with this book:

To Kristin Bonney, who started me on my Reiki journey and set me a good example to follow;

To William Lee Rand, who initiated me as a Master in Usui Reiki, Usui/Tibetan Reiki and Karuna Reiki®, and who encouraged me to always be myself in Reiki;

To Frank Arjava Petter and Chetna Kobayashi, for bringing the first translation of Usui's original Reiki manual to the West;

To Hiroshi Doi, and his students Andy Bowling and Ann Rogers, for their knowledge and experience of the original Japanese techniques;

To the Reiki Association, and to Light and Adonea, for the information about different forms of Reiki;

To the UK Reiki Federation, for the information on legal issues;

To the many spiritual teachers who have guided and inspired me, especially Gill Edwards, Karen Kingston, Mike Robinson, and Orin and DaBen;

To my friends and fellow Reiki Masters Carol and Mark Melling, Wendy Monks and the Rev. Simon John Barlow, for the inspirational example they set as people who really "walk their talk";

To my son, Chris, and daughter, Kathy, for their loving support and practical help;

And to all my Reiki students, for the love and learning they have brought me.

Contents

Part IV: The Japanese Tradition

Part V: More Steps Along the Reiki Path

Introduction

Reiki for Life is aimed at anyone interested in healing and self-healing with Reiki at any level, from absolute beginners to Practitioners and Masters. Unlike other books on Reiki, it is a complete guide to Reiki practice, giving all the Reiki techniques from the well-known Western tradition, including some never in print before. It also presents additional methods originally used by Dr. Mikao Usui, the founder of the Reiki healing system, which until recently were only available to Reiki students in Japan.

The book explores for the first time the true depth, power and promise of this wonderful healing system. From the development of Reiki in both Japan and the West to a comprehensive description of First and Second Degree techniques, it provides an essential resource for Reiki practice in the twenty-first century. It looks at the necessary background information about energy and meta-physical beliefs and provides a thorough foundation in the basics of self-treatment and how to treat others with Reiki at First Degree. However, it goes much further than other books: it emphasizes the holistic nature and spiritual aspects of Reiki and examines the personal and spiritual impact of becoming a Practitioner or a Master. It explains in detail how to carry out distant healing treatments and methods to heal and let go of personal problems as well as many other advanced techniques. In addition, it shows how the newly discovered Japanese techniques for energetic cleansing, healing and spiritual development can be used to enhance your practice of Reiki. Its aim, therefore, is to help anyone at any level to reach his or her full potential as a healing channel for Reiki.

There are traditionally three levels of qualification in Reiki. Reiki First Degree opens up the inner healing channel so that people can then use it for self-healing and healing others for the rest of their lives. At Reiki Second Degree three sacred symbols are taught, as well as some special techniques that intensify the Reiki and enable people to carry out effective distant (absent) healing, as well as other methods that promote deep healing of physical, mental and emotional problems. Reiki Third Degree is the level of a Reiki Master—someone who has committed his or her life to learning the mastery of Reiki, and who is qualified to teach others this amazing and powerful healing system.

Part I of the book begins by explaining what Reiki is and how it was discovered, and how it links with other energies in humans, animals, plants and the rest of the environment. It discusses the processes of healing from both conventional and traditional viewpoints, and provides comprehensive information about Reiki training, including what to expect from courses at each level.

Part II covers everything you need to know at Reiki First Degree, including methods for self-healing and how to carry out treatments on other people and animals, as well as some creative ways of using Reiki. In Part III there is a thorough explanation of the real impact and creative power of Second Degree, including how to use the Reiki symbols for self-healing and hands-on treatments of others, and how to carry out distant healing. A wide range of other advanced techniques is included, too, such as using Reiki to empower goals, heal emotional problems, create sacred space and protect yourself and those you care about.

Part IV introduces techniques only recently brought to the West from the Japanese Reiki traditions, including methods for self-cleansing and removing toxins from the body, as well as alternative ways of using the hands, such as patting and stroking, during Reiki treatments. The final section, Part V, looks at the importance of spiritual development with Reiki, and discusses what is needed to set up as a professional Practitioner, as well as how to become a Reiki Master.

Since the beginning of the 1990s, interest in complementary medicine and alternative therapies has increased tremendously.

Everywhere you look or listen there are television and radio programs and newspaper and magazine articles on holistic health and healing, and ways to improve your life physically, emotionally, psychologically and spiritually. For me the turning point was taking a course in Reiki, a hands-on healing technique that originated in Japan, and from that day in 1991 my life has changed for the better.

I began my journey of personal and spiritual discovery back in the 1970s with a growing interest in psychic abilities, but since that first Reiki course my main focus has been mind–body healing techniques and spiritual growth, although I have also developed skills as a clairvoyant and psychic channel. I worked for three years as a Reiki Practitioner before becoming a Reiki Master/Teacher of both the Usui Shiki Ryoho and Usui/Tibetan traditions in 1994, and a Karuna Reiki® Master/Teacher in 1996. In 2000 and 2003 I gained further experience and qualifications in the original techniques of Dr. Usui, the founder of the modern system of Reiki healing, which had only just been rediscovered after research into the Reiki traditions in Japan.

Over the past ten years or so I have continued to extend my knowledge and experience by studying a wide range of subjects, including meditation and visualization, NLP (neurolinguistic programing), kinesiology, metamorphic technique, Native American and contemporary shamanism, dowsing, feng shui and other topics that promote understanding, personal growth and a holistic view of the person. But my first love is, and always will be, Reiki.

My professional background and qualifications are in psychology, education and management, but in 1996 I gave up my career as a lecturer and senior manager at a college to enable myself to devote more time to teaching and writing books about Reiki. My first paperback, *An Introduction to Reiki*, was published by Piatkus in March 1999 (revised in 2007 as *The Basics of Reiki*).

I then began to realize that because the way Reiki training is carried out has changed significantly in recent years, many students were not able to get the best out of their use of Reiki, so I decided to write this second book. I chose the title for this book, *Reiki for Life*, for several reasons: first, because once you have acquired the ability to access Reiki healing energy, you retain that ability for the rest of your life. Second, because Reiki promotes healing and well-being for the whole person, it is definitely "for" an improved life. And third, the title reflects the fact that Reiki can potentially transform your life, as it stimulates personal and spiritual growth, encourages healthy changes in lifestyle, increases inspiration and intuition, and brings about realizations of our deeper, spiritual nature, which can be powerful and life-changing.

Until the late 1980s relatively few people were qualified to practice or teach Reiki, but during the 1990s there was an explosion of interest in all forms of healing, particularly in the West, and there are now probably several million people throughout the world who "have" Reiki—that is, they have acquired the ability to access this healing energy to help themselves and others.

The emphasis throughout *Reiki for Life* is on enjoying the healing and self-healing benefits of Reiki, and having fun being creative with it, while still treating it with the respect that it deserves as one of the world's most precious gifts for healing and spiritual growth. I wish you joy on your Reiki journey.

Part I

Simplicity and Power— Reiki Healing Energy

Chapter 1

The Discovery of Reiki

In this chapter we deal with what Reiki is and the meaning of the word *Reiki*, how, when and where Reiki was discovered, and how it has developed as a healing system both in the West and in Japan, where it originated.

WHAT IS REIKI?

Reiki is a safe, gentle, nonintrusive hands-on healing technique for use on yourself or with others, which uses spiritual energy to treat physical ailments without using pressure, manipulation or massage. However, it is much more than a physical therapy. It is a holistic system for balancing, healing and harmonizing all aspects of the person—body, mind, emotions and spirit—and it can also be used to encourage personal and spiritual awareness and growth.

THE WORD *REIKI*

The Japanese word *Reiki* (pronounced *Ray Kee*) is usually translated as "Universal Life-force Energy," or "God-directed Life-force Energy," or "Spiritual Energy." The word is divided into two parts:

Rei is translated as the "wisdom and knowledge of all the Universe" or "atmosphere of the Divine." It means the Higher Intelligence that guides the creation and functioning of the Universe; the wisdom that comes from God (or the Source, the Creator, the Universe or All That Is), which is all knowing, and which understands the need for and the cause of all problems and difficulties, and how to heal them.

Ki is the life-force energy that flows through every living thing—plants, animals and people—and that is present in some form in everything around us, even in rocks and inanimate objects.

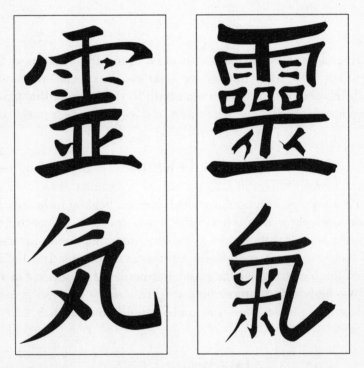

Modern Kanji for Rei Ki   **Older Kanji for Rei Ki**

Reiki is represented in the Japanese Kanji (Japanese alphabet) calligraphy in two slightly different ways. The image on the left is the more modern form, while that on the right is an older and more traditional way of writing the word Reiki.

In Japan the word *Reiki* can be used to describe any form of healing using spiritual energy, but in the West when we talk about

Reiki we are usually referring to the form of healing practice developed by a Japanese Buddhist priest, Dr. Mikao Usui (1865–1926), who, after many years of study, discovered a way of accessing and using this healing energy, and of passing this ability on to other people. During the last few years of his life he founded Usui Reiki Ryoho, which means the Usui Spiritual Energy Healing Method, and this has become widely known throughout the world as simply "Reiki."

HOW REIKI CAME TO THE WEST

Reiki as a healing system has been used and taught in the West since the late 1930s, and until the early 1990s the story of how Reiki was discovered was an oral history, handed down from teacher to student in a very traditional way. This story told that Dr. Mikao Usui was a learned scholar who taught in a Christian seminary. One day he was challenged by one of his students, who asked him if he believed in the Bible stories of Jesus's healing, and, if so, when were they going to be taught how to heal?

It was said that, as an honorable Japanese gentleman, upon realizing that he could not teach his students any healing techniques, he dedicated the rest of his life to finding out how Jesus and the Buddha had been able to heal. He was said to have traveled widely and learned other languages in order to research both Christian scriptures and Buddhist teachings, including Japanese and Sanskrit Sutras (sacred texts). He finally ended up in a Zen Buddhist monastery, where the Abbot advised him to meditate to find the answers he was seeking.

Then, at the end of a 21-day fasting retreat, Dr. Usui was apparently struck by a great light. He saw the sacred symbols he had earlier found during his research, and he acquired a deep understanding of them, receiving a spiritual empowerment (empower means "to give to" or "to enable," and a spiritual empowerment means to transfer wisdom, insight and ability by means of an inpouring of spiritual energy) and achieving enlightenment, a state of spiritual insight brought on by joining with and becoming one with the Light. When it was over, despite weakness after his long fast, he was able to rush down the mountain, but he injured his foot in his haste. When he bent down to hold his toe, he found that the bleeding had stopped, the pain had gone away and he was healed. Later he healed a young girl's toothache and his friend the Abbot's arthritis, so he came to realize that he had finally discovered the healing power for which he had been searching.

The story then told that he spent many years healing people in Japan before passing his knowledge and teachings on to Dr. Chujiro Hayashi (1879–1940), a naval commander. After Dr. Usui's death Hayashi was said to have opened a Reiki clinic. One day in 1935 a young woman from Hawaii named Hawayo Takata (1900–1980), who was visiting relatives in Japan, came to the clinic for treatment of a serious illness. She was so impressed with the success of her treatment that she begged to be able to learn Reiki, and Hayashi eventually agreed to teach her.

Takata lived with his family and worked without pay in his clinic in exchange for the privilege of being able to learn the first and second levels of this healing system. She returned to Hawaii in 1937 and opened the first Reiki clinic in the West, where Hayashi and his family visited her. He passed on the final level of the Reiki teachings to her in 1938 before he returned to Japan, so that she would be able to teach this healing art to others. The story Mrs. Takata told was that during World War II all of Hayashi's Reiki students in Japan were killed, and she was therefore the only Reiki teacher alive.

Mrs. Takata continued to teach Reiki and run her clinic in Hawaii, but also traveled extensively throughout the U.S. and Canada, treating people with Reiki and teaching them how to use Reiki for themselves. She held classes in two levels of Reiki training, which she called First Degree and Second Degree. However, it was the 1970s before she began to impart the final level of teachings, the Third Degree, which she called Reiki Master (a rough translation of "*Sensei*," meaning "respected teacher" in Japanese), so that others would be able to pass on the teachings when she had gone. By the time of her death in December 1980, after 42 years of teaching Reiki, she had trained the following 22 Masters, and it is through them that Reiki has spread so widely throughout the Western world:

George Araki
Dorothy Baba
Ursula Baylow
Rick Bockner
Patricia Bowling
Barbara Brown
Fran Brown
Phyllis Furumoto
Beth Gray
John Gray
Iris Ishikuro
Harru Kuboi
Ethel Lombardi
Barbara McCullough
Mary McFadyen
Paul Mitchell
Bethel Phaigh
Shinobu Saito
Virginia Samdahl
Wanja Twan
Barbara Weber Ray
Kay Yamashita

Mrs. Takata established a system of teaching Reiki that survives to this day, although in the last twenty years there have been several changes made by various Masters, which will be outlined in later chapters. She taught the system in three levels, as taught by Hayashi. However, she adapted the teaching to suit Western students, for example, teaching First Degree or Second Degree as workshops held over just a few days, rather than expecting students to work in her clinic for months. However, Master level was usually taught as a form of apprenticeship, working alongside Takata for perhaps a year.

Mrs. Takata used the ceremonial spiritual empowerment that Hayashi had taught her, which she called an initiation, to transfer the healing ability to her students. She also taught the four Reiki symbols. These are sacred shapes which alter the way Reiki can be used and which also increase its strength. Reiki treatments were carried out using a series of 12 basic hand positions, each held for five minutes, and she encouraged her students to treat themselves with Reiki every day. In addition, realizing that in the West her students related money to importance, and wanting people to value the incredible gift of Reiki, she charged high course fees—U.S. $150 for Reiki 1, $500 for Reiki 2, and $10,000 for Reiki 3. To put this into context, in the early 1970s when Takata began to teach Reiki Masters, $10,000 would buy a house in the United States.

THE DEVELOPMENT OF REIKI IN THE WEST

After Hawayo Takata's death, a group of her Masters met in Hawaii in 1982 to discuss how Reiki should progress, and who should become the next leader, or "Grand Master." It appears that there were two "favorites" for the post—Phyllis Lei Furumoto, Mrs. Takata's granddaughter, and Barbara Weber Ray. Phyllis agreed to follow in her grandmother's footsteps and was therefore elected by the majority of the Masters. Soon afterward Dr. Barbara Weber Ray broke away to found her own system of Reiki called The Radiance® Technique, which she later renamed Real Reiki®.

That historic first meeting in 1982 allowed Western Reiki Masters to share their experiences for the first time, and they discovered differences in the way they had been taught—perhaps because Mrs. Takata had taught the system as an oral tradition, not even allowing her student Masters to take notes. They made some decisions to standardize the system and these have had a major influence on the development of Reiki in the West, establishing what we now call the Western tradition of Reiki.

The Masters agreed on how the system should be taught and the exact form of each of the four Reiki symbols. They also adopted the same pricing structure Mrs. Takata had inaugurated. At a further meeting in British Columbia in 1983, The Reiki Alliance was formed. This is an organization of Reiki Masters who recognize Phyllis Lei Furumoto as the Grand Master, and whose purpose is to support each member as teachers of the Usui System of Reiki.

Until 1988, following the tradition that her grandmother had started, only Phyllis Furumoto, as Grand Master, was entitled to train other Masters, but in a gathering at Friedricksburg that year she announced that any suitably experienced Master could teach other Masters. This significant decision is what opened up Reiki in the West to the inevitable changes that result from expansion.

By the early 1990s the number of Masters and Practitioners had grown extensively, and an increasing number of Masters moved away from the system agreed on by the Reiki Alliance to work independently, changing the way Reiki was taught. Written manuals and books about Reiki began to appear, additional hand positions were used, extra symbols were added, and the time between levels was shortened, so that sometimes Reiki 1 and Reiki 2 were taught on two consecutive days.

The way the Master level was taught also changed considerably. Instead of an apprenticeship system, where one or two trainee Masters would work alongside an established Master for a year or more, the Reiki Third Degree began to be taught in large groups in courses lasting just a few days. Also, students were allowed to progress through the three levels very quickly—often within one year, and sometimes within only a few months or even weeks. This resulted in a massive expansion in the number of Masters, with a consequent growth in the number of people learning First and Second Degree Reiki, so that Reiki rapidly spread all over the world.

NEW INFORMATION ABOUT REIKI

In the late 1990s new information began to come to the West from Japan, which revealed that Dr. Usui had been a Buddhist priest, not a Christian priest, and that he had passed his complete teachings on to 17 people, not only to Chujiro Hayashi. It turned out that not all the Reiki Masters in Japan had been killed during World War II, and it became apparent that Reiki had continued to be taught there for the whole of the time since Dr. Usui's death. Indeed, an organization existed which was dedicated to preserving the original teachings of Dr. Usui—the Usui Reiki Ryoho Gakkai.

This fuller and more accurate picture of Reiki's discovery and development came particularly from two men—Frank Arjava Petter, a European Reiki Master living and working in Japan with his Japanese wife, Chetna Kobayashi, and Hiroshi Doi, a Japanese Reiki Master who has trained in both Japanese and Western Reiki traditions. Others who have contributed to our current knowledge of Japanese Reiki include Dave King, Melissa Riggall and Robert Jefford, all of whom have spent time researching in Japan.

THE BACKGROUND TO THE DISCOVERY OF REIKI

We now know that Dr. Usui was born in Taniai-mura (now Miyama-cho) in Japan on August 15, 1865, and that he began his study of

Buddhism at the age of four, when he was sent to a monastery school run by Tendai Buddhist monks. He studied martial arts from the age of 12, reaching the highest levels of Menkyo Kaiden by his mid-twenties and of other ancient Japanese systems as he got older, including Ki-Ko, the Japanese form of the Chinese martial art and energy balancing system known as chi kung. He also learned meditation and healing.

During his adult life Dr. Usui held many different jobs, including a government officer, a businessman, a journalist and secretary to the Mayor of Tokyo. For a while he is also said to have worked as a missionary (quoted on his memorial stone), although where and to what purpose is unclear, although it may refer to his prison work. However, as he lived a relatively normal life with a wife and children, it is unlikely that he was a cloistered monk. He is believed to have converted from Tendai to Shingon Buddhism by the time he was 27, and is known to have studied other forms of Buddhism from the Shinto and Mahayana (Mikkyo) sects. At the age of 53 he began a three-year training in Zen Buddhism.

As he grew up Usui was undoubtedly influenced by the expansiveness which was characteristic of the reign of Emperor Mutsuhito (known as the Meiji Emperor), who came to the throne when Usui was nearly three years old. During his reign, known as the Meiji Restoration period (1868–1912) a new wave of openness began as Japan's previously closed borders were opened for the first time in many centuries.

The country changed from an agrarian economy to an industrial one, and this resulted in an eagerness to explore the benefits of Western influences, with a consequent freedom for Japanese nationals to travel outside their own country. Many Japanese scholars were sent abroad to study Western languages and sciences, and Dr. Usui is known to have traveled widely, and to have pursued a life of study. It states on his memorial, situated in the graveyard of the Seihoji temple in Tokyo, that he visited China, the U.S. and Europe, and that he was fond of reading, acquiring knowledge of medicine, history, psychology and world religions.

As part of his training in Zen Buddhism Usui would have been working toward achieving *Satori*, the state of Spiritual Enlightenment. His memorial confirms that he had an experience of mystical enlightenment on Mount Kurama, near Kyoto. Early 1922 is the most probable date, since this follows his entry into Zen Buddhism in 1918, although several Japanese books give the date as 1914. Apparently after advice from his Zen Master, he decided to undergo *shyu gyo*, a strict spiritual discipline involving meditation and fasting for 21 days, until he either died or became enlightened. On the last morning of his fast he experienced "a great Reiki over his head" (quoted on Usui's memorial), which enabled him to become enlightened, and to acquire the ability to access healing energy (Reiki) and to pass that ability on to others.

Dr. Usui then spent the few years before his death on March 9, 1926, at the age of 60 practicing and teaching his healing system— Usui Reiki Ryoho, or the Usui Spiritual Energy Healing Method— during which time he passed on his knowledge to others so that the teachings could continue. His memorial states: "If Reiki can be spread throughout the world it will touch the human heart and the morals of society. It will be helpful for many people, not only healing disease, but the Earth as a whole." His wishes have come true, perhaps even beyond what he could have envisaged, and there are now millions of people around the world using Reiki.

THE DEVELOPMENT OF REIKI IN JAPAN

It is a facet of Japanese culture that knowledge or important information is normally kept secret (or sacred, as the words are synonymous in the Japanese language) within family groups, which is the main reason why it has taken so long for accurate information to come to the West about Reiki's development.

Initially Dr. Usui is believed to have used Reiki only on himself and his family, and it is reported that Reiki cured his wife of a serious illness at that time. However, so important did he realize his discovery to be that he decided to begin teaching people how to access this healing energy, and he made *Sho-den* (the first level of Reiki training) "freely available to all of the people"—a direct quote from one of his teaching manuals, the *Usui Reiki Hikkei*.

There is reliable information, provided on Usui's memorial, that about 2,000 people learned Reiki from Dr. Usui (which he also called *Teate*, meaning "healing hands"), but most of these would only have achieved the first level of training, *Sho-den* (meaning "the

entrance"), equivalent to First Degree in the West. It appears that
between 30 and 50 people may have learned the second level, *Oku-
den* (meaning "the deep inside"), equivalent to the Western Second
Degree, but not more than 17 acquired the third level, *Shinpi-den*
(meaning "the mystery/secret teachings"), which is what we call
Third Degree, or Reiki Master. They included five Buddhist nuns,
four naval officers and eight other men, but little else is known
about them, despite the fact that all of Dr. Usui's students who
achieved *Oku-den* and *Shinpi-den* were recorded with the Education
Departments in Japan. However, some of these records may have
been lost in the earthquake which affected Tokyo in 1925. The
following ten are listed:

Juzaburo Ushida (rear admiral)
Kan'ichi Takatomi (rear admiral)
Tetsutaro Imaizumi (rear admiral)
Chujiro Hayashi (admiral)
Haru Nagao (occupation
  unknown)
Toshihiro Eguchi (school-
  teacher)

Yoshiharu Watanabe
  (philosopher)
Sono'o Tsuboi (tea ceremony
  Master)
Imae Mine (musician)
Masayuki Okada (author of
  the inscription on
  Dr. Usui's memorial)

In April 1922 Dr. Usui opened his first clinic in Harajuku, Tokyo,
where he practiced and taught Reiki. His healing skills must have
been extraordinary, as he was renowned all over Japan, and
admired as "the pioneer of restarting Hands-on Healing from past
generations" (a quote from his memorial), and the number of
people helped by Reiki is reported to have been several hundred
thousand, including many of those injured in the Tokyo earthquake on September 1, 1923—although this number must have
included people helped by Dr. Usui's students, as well as those
helped by him personally! (Usui became well known for this work
and was apparently praised by the then-emperor, Taisho.)

The emphasis of Dr. Usui's teaching was as much about a
spiritual awakening as on purely physical healing. The importance
of self-healing was therefore imparted, as well as the benefits of
living a "proper" life, using the Reiki principles as a foundation,
which he adopted from the Meiji Emperor. Below is a version of
these principles that comes from an original document written in
Dr. Usui's own handwriting (in Japanese Kanji), which has now

been translated and appears in Frank Arjava Petter's book *The Legacy of Dr. Usui*:

Shoufuku no hihoo	**The secret method of inviting happiness**
Manbyo no ley-yaku	The wonderful medicine for all diseases (of the body and the soul)
Kyo dake wa	Just today:
1. *Okoru-na*	1. Do not get angry
2. *Shimpai suna*	2. Do not worry
3. *Kansha shite*	3. Show appreciation
4. *Goo hage me*	4. Work hard (on yourself)
5. *Hito ni shinsetsu ni*	5. Be kind to others
Asa yuu Gassho shite, koko-ro ni nenji, Kuchi ni tonaeyo	Mornings and evenings, sit in the *Gassho* position and repeat these words out loud and in your heart. ("*Gassho*" means to sit quietly with your hands together in the prayer position, with your thumbs pointing to the center of your chest.)
Shin shin kaizen, Usui Reiki Ryoho	(For the) improvement of body and soul, Usui Spiritual Energy Healing Method
Chosso Usui Mikao	The founder, Mikao Usui

In addition, Dr. Usui used 125 inspirational poems (*Gyosei*) from the Meiji Emperor Mutsuhito as a guide to his students in their personal and spiritual development. Here is one example of the stylized *Waka* (also called *Tanka*) poetry written by Emperor Mutsuhito which Dr. Usui taught to his students:

The Wave
One moment stormy
The next it is calm
The wave in the ocean
Is actually
Just like the human existence.

All 125 Waka poems are given in *Spirit of Reiki*, by Walter Lubeck, Frank Arjava Petter and William Rand.

He incorporated other aspects of his many years of Buddhist and martial arts training into his Reiki teaching, including meditation, self-cleansing and a simple but powerful method of spiritual empowerment called *Rei-ju*, as well as some Shinto and Ki-Ko energy practices. It seems that he worked intuitively on people, placing one or both hands wherever he detected energy imbalances that seemed in need of healing.

Once he began to teach others to do Reiki he found that instructions were needed, and he wrote the *Usui Reiki Hikkei*, which was a manual to be given to his students. Frank Arjava Petter and his wife, Chetna Kobayashi, have translated a copy of Dr. Usui's manual (*The Original Reiki Handbook of Dr. Mikao Usui*, by Frank Arjava Petter, Lotus Press, 1999), and it gives instructions for the treatment of particular illnesses and parts of the body using specific combinations from the total list of almost 70 hand positions.

THE FOUNDING OF THE USUI REIKI RYOHO GAKKAI

Mikao Usui is also credited with founding the Usui Reiki Ryoho Gakkai (meaning the Usui Reiki Healing Method Learning Society), an organization dedicated to keeping the Reiki teachings alive, although it is possible that his followers started it after his death, naming Dr. Usui as the founder as a mark of respect. This society has continued to practice and teach Reiki uninterrupted since 1926, the first few leaders being *Shinpi-den* students taught by Dr. Usui. They do not take the title of Grand Master, but are simply referred to as presidents of the society, and they are listed as:

1. Mikao Usui   5. Hoichi Wanami
2. Juzaburo Ushida   6. Mrs. Kimiko Koyama
3. Kan'ichi Taketomi   7. Masayoshi Kondo (from 1999)
4. Yoshiharu Watanabe

The Gakkai members follow Dr. Usui's teachings very closely, and they have in their possession two manuals produced by Dr. Usui (the *Usui Reiki Hikkei*). One of these contains an explanation of his energy healing method, the *Usui Reiki Ryoho*, and the other gives details of the various healing techniques, including specific hand positions for different diseases and physical problems, as mentioned above.

The Gakkai holds regular meetings in Tokyo and elsewhere in Japan for their members, where the students sing *Waka* poetry, chant the Reiki Principles and do *Hatsurei-ho* (a combined meditation and cleansing practice); each time they attend they receive a *Rei-ju* empowerment from one of the six *Shinpi-den* members, for cleansing, purification and to strengthen their ability to access Reiki.

CURRENT ISSUES WITHIN THE REIKI COMMUNITY

For a number of years questions have been asked about why the story Mrs. Takata told about the rediscovery of Reiki became Christianized, but this may well have been because both during and after World War II she was training people in the U.S. in a Japanese technique based on Buddhist teachings. Perhaps without introducing the idea that Dr. Usui was a Christian priest, things might have become very awkward for her.

We now realize that it would have been very unlikely for Dr. Usui to train as a Christian priest, because Christianity was banned in Japan until 1873, well after Dr. Usui began his Buddhist training. No record can be found of Dr. Usui's attending or teaching at any of the Japanese or U.S. colleges or universities that Mrs. Takata included in her story (my Reiki Master, William Lee Rand, has letters from each of the institutions confirming that no record of Mikao Usui can be found as either a student or teacher).

When in the late 1990s information came out of Japan about a range of techniques that did not seem to have been taught in the West through the Takata lineage—for example, the *Hatsurei-ho*, a meditation and self-cleansing technique, or alternative ways of using the hands during treatments, such as *Oshi-te Chiryo-ho*, tapping with the fingertips (see Chapter 16)—there was confusion, even indignation, in the Reiki community. Some people wanted to reject the new information, and stick to what they already knew, while others wanted to throw out all they had learned in the West, and use only the techniques from the Japanese traditions. Others were angry that they had been denied the chance of learning these valuable methods, and were critical of the Western lineage.

The spirit of Reiki training in the West was probably originally very similar to that in Japan. However, it seems possible that Mrs. Takata did teach many of what we now know were Dr. Usui's original methods, although she did not use their Japanese names. Some methods were seemingly only taught to Masters. Perhaps because the Masters she trained were not allowed to take notes, they simply forgot, or they did not realize the importance of some of the techniques because they did not come from a Buddhist background, where the spiritual and energetic significance of each method would have been more obvious.

EXPLORING THE DIFFERENCES

We know that in Japan the numbering of the levels is reversed, so what we would refer to as the first level, *Sho-den*, equivalent to our First Degree, is actually their sixth degree, which is itself divided into four parts: *Loku-To* (Sixth Degree), *Go-To* (Fifth Degree), *Yon-To* (Fourth Degree) and *San-To* (Third Degree). This is probably why we have four attunements in the traditional Western system of teaching Reiki.

Sho-den can be learned by anyone, but the second level, *Oku-den*, which is divided into two parts, *Okuden-Zenki* when the symbols are taught, and *Okuden-Koko* when distant and mental healing methods are taught, is only given when a student can demonstrate that they are accessing an appropriate amount of Reiki healing energy, and are proficient in the techniques, which may take ten years or more.

Students are expected to practice Reiki daily, to obey the five Principles and to make an effort to live those principles in their daily lives, encouraging mental and emotional growth and development. They are also expected to practice *Hatsurei-ho* daily, for self-cleansing and spiritual enhancement, and to continue their spiritual development, partly by attending regular training seminars where they receive *Rei-ju* attunements.

Receiving these regular *Rei-ju* attunements helps students develop their intuitive skills so that they become better able to detect and treat physical illnesses. This process is called *Byosen*, which is being able to feel energy from a source of illness, and being able to judge a symptom and the number of days of healing that will be required; or *Reiji*, where the hands go intuitively to affected areas and start sending Reiki. Very few people in Japan ever reach the advanced level of *Shinpi-den*, the equivalent of a Western Reiki Master, even after many, many years of practice.

Reiki has developed differently in the West, perhaps because we have not had the same spiritual background or the cultural under-standing of energies resulting in the need for a self-cleansing tradition. Although some Masters did bring their students together regularly to practice Reiki, no *Rei-ju* empowerments were given, because these were unknown to us until 1999. There has also been less emphasis on developing sensitivity in the hands with Reiki, which probably accounts for the system we have of 12 or more hand positions being held for five minutes each. This enables the Reiki to flow everywhere in the body, so that each person can receive the Reiki wherever they need it.

Since Mrs. Takata's death many Masters have chosen to change the way Reiki is taught, so that there are now more than 30 different types of Reiki being practiced in the West. Some are based very closely on Takata's system, while others have introduced many new "channeled" (receiving insight from spiritual sources) symbols, different attunement procedures and other practices, and no doubt more will appear in the future. However, now that we have discovered Dr. Usui's original techniques these can be integrated into Reiki practice, so we have even more tools available to us.

The aim of this book is to show the enormous potential of integrating these two healing systems, whose roots are firmly based in Eastern philosophy and wisdom, but whose body is expanding with the collected wisdom of many Western and Japanese Masters and Practitioners. In the next chapter we look in more depth at Reiki as a healing energy, and at its relationship to other energies such as those that comprise the human energy body.

Chapter 2

Reiki and Energy

Reiki is an energy—as explained in the last chapter, the word means spiritual energy or universal life-force energy. When we use it in healing, it acts holistically, affecting all of the energies that comprise the human body or animals or anything else in the natural world. To make later sections easier to understand, I want to first introduce energy in a wider context, especially electromagnetic energy, because this is what makes up our physical body as well as the energy field that surrounds and interpenetrates it.

ENERGY IS ALL THERE IS

We talk about "energy" in different ways, perhaps referring to energy sources such as coal, gas, wind power or electricity, or the caloric value of food, but the definition of energy is much broader than that. Einstein and later quantum physicists have explained that at an atomic level everything that exists in the Universe is energy, vibrating and oscillating at different rates; that physical matter and energy are just two forms of the same thing. So energy is all there is. We are familiar with some of these energetic vibrations, such as sound, light, radio waves and X-rays. These are all part of the electromagnetic spectrum, and from a scientific perspective the only difference between these various forms of energy is that each oscillates at a different frequency or rate of vibration.

Human beings are also comprised of electromagnetic energy, and every cell, atom and subatomic particle that makes up the human body is vibrating at different rates depending upon their biochemical makeup. For example, the specific electrical output of the human heart can be measured on an ECG machine (electrocardiogram). Also, the electromagnetic output of the whole body can be measured using an electromyograph, and the normal biological frequency for the human body is around 250 cps (cycles per second). However, some research that is very relevant to our understanding of human energy was carried out on a variety of people, recording the output at sites on the body traditionally associated with high-energy spots known as chakras (from the Sanskrit word for wheel or vortex), and some very interesting results were obtained.

Most people in the study recorded the normal range, around 250 cps, but when the tests were carried out on people who used healing energies (such as Reiki) and others who actively used their psychic ability, it was found that their frequencies registered in a band between 400 and 800 cps. Even higher frequencies—more than 900 cps—were found in people who were described as "mystical personalities."

These people were not only psychics and healers, but also followed a very spiritual path and were able to meditate deeply; moreover, they felt a connection to everything in nature and beyond, and held holistic and metaphysical beliefs. As you will see in later chapters, when I talk about Reiki "raising your vibrations," there is now scientific evidence to prove that's true.

But what is interesting is that science has finally confirmed something that has been part of the spiritual wisdom of many cultures for thousands of years—that an unseen energy flows through and connects all living things. This energy has various names, depending upon the culture or spiritual tradition, probably the most commonly known being *Ki* (Japanese) and *Chi* or *Qi* (Chinese), but it can also be referred to as *Prana* (Indian), Light or Spirit or the Holy Ghost (Christian), or as Vitality or Life force. As this book is about Reiki I will refer to it by its Japanese name, *Ki*, or as life force, but before we examine Reiki's connection to this life-force energy in more detail, I want to explain the human energy body in greater depth.

The Human Energy Body

The physical body is something we all know about—we can see it and feel it—yet every cell in it is still energy or light, vibrating at a slow enough rate to make it into visible physical matter. However, surrounding and interpenetrating our physical body is another body of energy, this time made up of much finer and lighter vibrations, which is most commonly called the aura, the auric field or the human energy body.

This auric field is as much a part of you as your physical body— indeed, your physical body is really just the densest inner layer of this flowing energy field. However, the higher frequencies of the energies that make up the aura mean that it is harder to see with the naked eye, although it can be detected by some scientific equipment, and can also be photographed using a specially developed Kirlian camera. Each person's energy body has its own distinctive energy signature—its energetic vibrational frequencies are unique, just as fingerprints are unique to each individual.

In addition to the aura, our energy body contains some energy centers known as chakras and a range of energy channels flowing through the body called meridians. Perhaps the easiest way of understanding this is to think of your energy body in similar terms to your physical body. The aura is the energy equivalent of your whole physical body, the chakras are equivalent to your brain and major organs, and the meridians are similar to your veins and arteries, but instead of blood, they carry energy—*Ki*—all over the body.

The Aura

This is a field of energy or light that completely surrounds the physical body above, below and on all sides. It is made up of seven layers, with the inner layers closest to the physical body being comprised of the densest energy, and each succeeding layer being of finer and higher vibrations. Most people have an oval (elliptical) aura, which is slightly larger at the back than at the front, and fairly narrow at the sides, and it also stretches above the head and below the feet. A person's aura is not always the same size—it can expand or contract depending upon a variety of factors such as how healthy you are, how you are feeling emotionally or psychologically at any given moment, or how comfortable you feel with the people who are in your immediate surroundings.

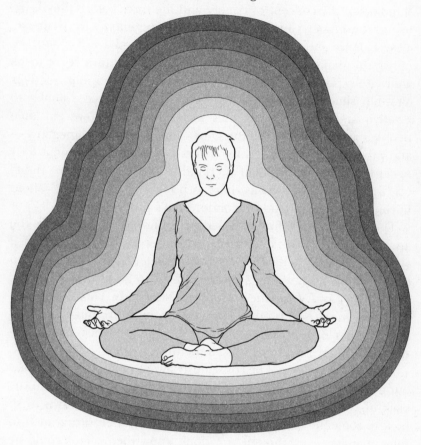

The seven layers of the aura.

This aura is spiritual energy that is present from birth (and possibly before) until death. After physical death, no aura can be detected, because the life force no longer exists. However, in a living person the outer edges and the individual layers of the aura can be detected using dowsing rods or a pendulum, and can also be sensed with the hands. The densest layers, nearest the body, can also be seen with the naked eye with a little practice. Painters over the centuries have depicted the aura around the heads of angels, saints and prophets as a bright golden halo, indicating their pure and spiritual energy.

Detecting auras is the first thing I teach in my Reiki classes. Apart from being great fun it also allows people to gain a real understanding of the concept of energy and life force before they learn to use the higher vibrations of Reiki healing energy to permeate, clear, balance and energize the whole energy body.

For the majority of people, the layers of the aura seem to be alternately positive and negative energy—not meaning good or bad, but simply indicating a different set of vibrations, similar to positive and negative polarities in magnetism. However, some people's auric layers are all the same—all positive, or all negative— and others have the first three layers positive, and the next four negative and so on. Each person is individual, so there is no "right" or "wrong" in this—just as there is no "right" or "wrong" about having dark hair instead of blonde. That's just the way it is.

The biggest shock for most people is finding out how large the aura can be. Of course it varies from person to person, and it changes from day to day anyway, but the outer layer of the aura can be anywhere from about 2 meters (6½ ft) to 20 meters (66 ft) or even farther away from the person's physical body. This means that, whenever we are with other people, our auras are intermingling, and whether or not we are mindful of it we are "picking up" signals from other people's auras all the time.

Although we may not be consciously aware of the fact, we all use our auras as sensing devices—what you might call "the eyes in the back of your head." Have you ever felt particularly drawn to sit next to someone or felt a sense of discomfort when sitting next to someone else, even though you don't know them? This could be because your aura has already "picked up" either complementary or disturbing energies within the other person's aura.

Or have you ever experienced a strange prickling sensation at the back of your neck when someone has been looking at you from behind? Perhaps you have been able to sense the atmosphere within in a room before you have even opened the door? Not surprising, really, when you consider that your aura may extend 10 or more meters (30 or more feet) ahead of you, so that it is already in the room picking up the vibrations of other people's auric fields; this is because the finer and lighter vibrations of auric energy can pass through the denser energy of physical matter.

The Chakras

Chakra is a Sanskrit word meaning wheel or vortex, and there are seven major chakras in the human energy body located at (1) the base of the spine/perinium, (2) near the navel, (3) at the solar plexus, (4) in the middle of the chest, (5) in the throat, (6) in the center of the brow and (7) at the crown of the head. In addition there are more than 20 minor chakras, for example, in the palms of the hands, on the knees and on the soles of the feet. A healthy chakra can be seen psychically vibrating evenly in a circular motion, resembling a funnel that is fairly narrow close to the body, but that becomes wider as it gets farther away.

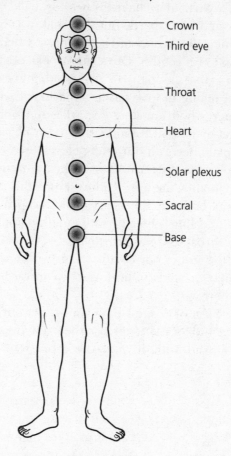

The seven major chakras.

Chakras are an essential part of our body's energy system, because they are intimately connected with our physical health. Each is linked with specific parts of the body and to systems within the body. You will see in later chapters that when carrying out a Reiki treatment, either on yourself or on another person, your hands are placed near the major chakras, as this is where life-force energy—and Reiki—can be most easily absorbed, transformed and distributed throughout the physical and energy bodies. It is also possible to become sensitive enough to "read" our own or others' energy bodies so that the Reiki healing energy can be directed into those areas that need it.

When a particular chakra is healthy, balanced and open, so are its connected body parts, but if a chakra is blocked, damaged or closed, then the health of the connected body parts and systems will begin to reflect this. Our chakras, like our aura, are affected by everything that happens to us—good things as well as bad. For example, falling in love has an amazingly beneficial effect on our whole energy body, making it sparkle and zing with color, whereas emotional or mental traumas, and even negative words, can have detrimental effects on our energy levels.

When we use the term "broken heart" to describe the feeling of devastation after the loss of a loved one, this is actually reflected in the energy body, as the heart chakra appears to have breaks or tears in it. Feeling "choked" with emotion appears as imbalances in both the throat and the heart chakras; the sacral chakra, near our navel, is the seat of our creativity, so "writer's block" might show as a dark mist or spots indicating obstruction in the natural flow of energy there.

In the chart opposite I have shown not only each chakra's number, name and location, but also the color vibration, body parts and systems linked with it, and the aspects of our lives associated with it.

Chakra Number	Chakra	Location	Color	Body Parts/ Systems	Associated Life Aspects
7	Crown (*sahasrara*)	Top of head	Violet, purple or white	Pineal, nervous system, mind and whole body	Enlightenment, knowledge, spirituality, understanding, self-realization, unity, connection, fulfillment, completion, mysticism, universal consciousness *I know*
6	Brow or third eye (*ajna*)	Center of forehead	Indigo	Pituitary, brain, hypothalamus, endocrine system, head, eyes, face	Clairvoyance, intuition, insight, imagination, spiritual awareness, vision, individual consciousness, *I see*
5	Throat (*vishuddha*)	Throat	Blue	Thyroid, parathyroid, metabolism, ears, nose, mouth, teeth, neck, throat	Communication, creativity, self-expression, abundance, sound, vibration, receiving *I speak*
4	Heart (*anahata*)	Center of chest (sternum)	Green or pink	Thymus, respiration, circulation, immune system, heart, lungs, upper back, arms, hands	Unconditional love, balance, unity, compassion, kindness, affinity, giving, limitless, infinite *I love*
3	Solar plexus (*manipura*)	Solar plexus	Yellow	Pancreas, muscles, digestive system, liver, spleen, small intestine, gallbladder, middle back	Personal power, autonomy, will, purpose, control, self-determination, self-empowerment, energy, self-esteem, intellect, destiny *I can*

Chakra Number	Chakra	Location	Color	Body Parts/ Systems	Associated Life Aspects
2	Sacral (*svadhisthara*)	Abdomen (navel)	Orange	Testes/ovaries, reproductive system, uterus, sexuality, food, lower digestive organs, kidneys, prostate, urinary tract, lower back	Relationships, emotions, intimacy, sharing, sensations, appetite, pleasure, movement, imagination, the unconscious *I feel*
1	Root or base (*muladhara*)	Base of spine/ perineum	Red	Adrenals, skeleton, skin, blood, large intestine, pelvis, hips, legs, feet, elimination system	Survival, security, trust, grounding, physical body, money, home, job, sense of belonging, nature, biology, earth *I have*

The Meridians

Meridians are the final component of the human energy body, and the easiest way to describe them is that they are the energy equivalent of the arteries and veins that carry our blood around our bodies. Meridians are the channels that carry our life force, or *Ki*, around our body, and the major meridians route the energy longitudinally through the body, connecting with all of the body's major organs, but there are other smaller meridians (*nadis*) that crisscross throughout the body, connecting all the parts together so that *Ki* can flow everywhere.

It is on these Meridians that the various points exist that are used in complementary therapies such as acupuncture or acupressure, or that connect all parts of the body with the areas on the feet and hands used in reflexology.

THE HUMAN ENERGY BODY AND HEALTH

The state of the energy body is a very important element in the health of any individual, because if blockages and damage in the aura are not cleared and healed, they can eventually manifest themselves as physical illness or disease. Everything that happens to us affects the aura, whether they be negative or positive experiences, although of course it is the negative experiences that create the blockages and eventual damage.

Every negative thought you have ever had, every negative word you have spoken, will have had an effect on your aura and whole energy body, although these effects would normally only be lasting if the negative thoughts and words were consistently repeated. Similarly, any negative words spoken to you, or negative actions performed against you, can potentially form damaging energy patterns in your aura, particularly if they evoke your emotions.

Even reading the newspapers, which are usually filled with negative news, or watching violent or horror movies or television programs, has a dampening effect on your energy field. All of these things will lower your energy body's vibrations, or life force, but fortunately we are able to take in more life force, or *Ki*, every day, and thankfully our lives are not normally filled only with negative experiences.

The positive experiences we have—the love and affection from our family and friends, watching children at play, viewing a beautiful sunset, the satisfaction of a creative project or success at work—all contribute to raising our vibrations, or *Ki*, so the effects balance out for much of the time. It is therefore only major traumas and significant negative experiences that have the opportunity to damage our energy field beyond our normal ability to replenish and repair it.

The Role of *Ki*—Life-force Energy

Knowledge that our bodies are filled with life-force energy—*Ki*—and that this is directly connected to the quality of our health, has been part of the wisdom of many cultures for thousands of years, and has resulted in the development of many different forms of "energy medicine." Some of these require direct physical contact with the body, such as acupuncture, shiatsu and reflexology, while others are taken into the body in various forms, such as herbal, homeopathic and flower remedies.

Of course it is not only people who have energy bodies. All animals, birds, fish, insects and plants have detectable auras and, indeed, so do what we might term "inanimate" objects, such as rocks, crystals, minerals, metals and water.

The amount of *Ki* or life force within you varies from day to day—there is a natural rhythmic ebb and flow in the energies within our bodies—but we absorb *Ki* in various ways in order to "top up" our supply of life force, as we naturally use some each day. We absorb some in the form of food and drink—remember, all animal and plant life, and even water, is filled with *Ki* too—and we also take in *Ki* from the air we breathe and absorb it through our auric fields. *Ki* energy is everywhere; it is the connective force of the Universe so there is a limitless supply.

The levels of life force in our bodies have an impact on our inherent healing ability, as *Ki* helps to nourish the structure, organs and systems of the body, supporting them in their vital functions and contributing to the healthy growth and renewal of cells. However, the amount we absorb is not constant, and can depend on many factors, so we don't always sufficiently replenish our supply of *Ki*.

If this happens over some time our energy body can become too depleted, and this is when we become weaker and more susceptible to illness, the aging process and even physical death, because our *Ki*, or life force, is what defines us as living beings. Without it we would not be alive.

This means that when our *Ki* is high and flowing freely around our whole energy body, we feel healthy, strong, fit and full of energy. We also feel confident, ready to enjoy life and take on its challenges, and are much less likely to become ill. However, if our *Ki* is low, or if there is a restriction or blockage in its flow, we feel weak, tired, listless and lethargic, and are much more vulnerable to illness or "dis-ease."

REIKI AS AN ENERGY

The difference between *Ki* (life-force energy) and Reiki (spiritual energy, or universal life-force energy) is:

- *Ki* is the energy that surrounds and permeates everything.
- **Reiki** is a specific band or frequency of energy for healing and self-healing that works synergistically with *Ki*, but at a higher vibration. Reiki comes directly from the Source (or God, the

Creator, All That Is) and is directed by that Higher Intelligence for healing (or wholing) anything, whether animate or inanimate.

Because Reiki energy is vibrating at a very high rate it is not normally visible to the human eye, but its use can be detected by a Kirlian camera, and some people do see it, usually as a white/ gold stream of energy similar to the spiral shape of the DNA double helix. However, unlike *Ki*, which is present everywhere and in everything, Reiki does not flow automatically through everyone from birth. It flows only through people who have been "attuned" to its vibrational frequency. This attunement, or spiritual empowerment, is the way in which the healing ability of Reiki is passed energetically from a Reiki Master to a student during a sacred ceremony, which is a vital part of a Reiki course or workshop.

Connecting with Reiki Energy—the Spiritual Empowerment

In Buddhism a spiritual empowerment is a familiar but very special element in spiritual practice, and it is where wisdom, existential knowledge, insight and ability are passed from the Master by thought and intention deep into the student's mind, body and spirit. You may remember that Dr. Usui received a spiritual empowerment on Mount Kurama, where he achieved a deep knowledge and understanding of the Reiki symbols, and acquired the ability to heal.

The spiritual empowerment that is carried out by a Reiki Master is similar in nature, but less powerful, since Dr. Usui received the whole understanding and the full strength of Reiki in one single empowerment from the Highest Source, which also allowed him to become enlightened. As he had been involved in spiritual practice for about 50 years by that time, he was no doubt energetically far better prepared for such a tremendous experience and vast amount of healing energy than any of us would be.

In Usui Reiki there are a number of spiritual empowerments spread out between the various levels, so that the student has time to "acclimatize" to the levels of energy involved. We usually call these sacred ceremonies initiations or attunements, as they "initiate" the student into a new life with Reiki (initiate means to begin)

and "attune" the student to the unique vibrations of the Reiki spiritual healing energy (attune means to bring into harmony with).
The attunement sets up an energetic channel in the student,
through which the Reiki energy can flow from the Source, through
the student's energy body—the crown, brow, throat and heart
chakras—and out through the hands.

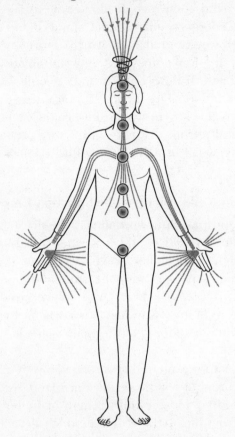

The flow of Reiki after attunement.

In effect, this attunement "reopens" an existing channel within
our energy body to our enlightened selves—our Soul/Spirit/Higher
Self—that part of us that is always and completely connected to
the Source/God/All That Is. While the Reiki may appear to come
from outside ourselves, entering through the crown chakra, this
only seems that way because we have a limited awareness of our
whole existence, and cannot "see" the full extent and potential of

our being, our Soul/Spirit/Higher Self, extending way beyond the confines of our physical bodies.

The "spiritual empowerment," which takes place during the attunement, is just that: it empowers a part of our spirit, Reiki, which we did not consciously know how to access before, so that we become aware of it for the first time. As soon as students have received this attunement they are able to access and use Reiki healing energy for themselves or to treat others. They will continue to be able to do so for the rest of their lives, as this healing energy comes through our Higher Selves, channeled from an inexhaustible source—God/Creator/All That Is/The Universe—whenever we want it to.

This "instant" acquisition of healing ability is one of the things that makes Reiki unique, but is probably also the most puzzling aspect of it to Western minds. We are not accustomed to anything so valuable being achieved so effortlessly, yet in the East spiritual empowerments are a well-known and accepted way of acquiring energy, knowledge, wisdom or insight. However, although Reiki may have its roots in Eastern spiritual practices, it is not a religion, so it can be made available to anyone, regardless of their personal beliefs. Also, Reiki does not depend on a person's intellectual capacity or level of spiritual development, so people of all ages and from all backgrounds can acquire the ability to channel Reiki healing energy simply and easily by attending a Reiki First Degree class and receiving the attunement. No specialized knowledge or skills are required, so Reiki is a very accessible way of learning how to help yourself and others.

REIKI ENERGY AS A HEALING TREATMENT

After an attunement a student can use Reiki on themselves or on other people. Many people who train in Reiki go on to become Practitioners or therapists, offering Reiki treatments in their own homes or natural health centers and even in some hospitals and clinics. The process of a Reiki healing treatment is very simple, and the person receiving it will usually either lie on a massage table or sit in a chair, and they can remain fully clothed, although they are usually asked to remove their shoes.

When people who have been attuned wish to use Reiki, they do not need to go through any complicated ritual—simply intending to use Reiki starts it flowing into their energy body, as shown in the illustration on page 30, and out through the palms of their hands. The Practitioner then places their hands very gently on specific places on the head and body of the person who wishes to receive a Reiki treatment, and either holds them still, or occasionally taps gently with the fingertips or pats lightly with the flat of the palm, so there is no need for massage or pressure of any kind. (More information on hand placements is included in chapters 6 and 7.)

Because Reiki is a very high vibrational energy, it can flow into, over and through anything, including solid matter. This enables it to work holistically on the whole person—chakras and aura, body and mind-consciousness, emotions and spirit. As Reiki flows into our aura and physical body, it helps to break down energetic disruptions or blockages, clearing and balancing the chakras and straightening the energy pathways (meridians) to allow the life-force to flow in a healthy and natural way around the whole body.

This influx of high-frequency healing energy stimulates and accelerates the body's own natural healing ability, so that pain relief and physical healing can take place quickly and easily—sometimes at quite extraordinary speed. Also, because Reiki is guided by a Higher Intelligence, it can make its way to those areas of the physical body and energy body that are most in need of healing, without any conscious direction from either the healer or the recipient. In addition, Reiki automatically adjusts to suit the recipient, so that each person receives as much or as little as they need, at an appropriate rate of flow.

Reiki acts to heal, harmonize and balance the whole self, and as it is guided by a higher wisdom and always works for the highest good of the person receiving it, it cannot be harmful in any way. The potential for healing with Reiki is unlimited, so anything can be treated, but it is important to rid yourself of specific expectations of what it will do, and how fast it will perform.

Many physical symptoms can be eased very quickly, while others may need lots of Reiki before starting to respond. However, it is essential to remember that it is a person's own body—either your own, if you are self-treating, or a client's if you are treating someone else—that is actually doing the healing, as you will see in the next chapter. Occasionally people report amazing, even miraculous, effects from Reiki treatments, while some gain partial or complete relief from symptoms for a time, and others experience little obvious effect.

Reiki is not a guaranteed "cure-all," because "healing" is not always the same as "curing." Healing does not always occur on the physical level first. Because Reiki works holistically and is guided by a Higher Intelligence, it may be that healing needs to happen first at the emotional level, with the releasing of anger, guilt or hatred, or it may be required first at the mental level, releasing negative thoughts, concepts or attitudes, before the physical symptoms can be addressed. Also, healing is a very personal issue, and if ten people displaying identical physical symptoms were given Reiki, there would be ten potentially different outcomes, because their mental, emotional and spiritual states would not be the same.

Ultimately, if the healing is to be permanent you have to take responsibility for healing the cause. This may mean changing how you think or the way you relate to other people, or even altering your whole lifestyle, from your diet and home environment to your close relationships and your job or career. However, when Reiki flows through you it can help with these adjustments too, allowing you to approach the changes in a calm, relaxed and accepting state of mind.

In the next chapter we take a broad look at healing, and at why people become ill, as well as at the role Reiki can play in achieving health and well-being.

Chapter 3

Healing and Wholing

Healing is described in the dictionary as "to be restored to health; to repair by natural processes, as by scar formation; to cure," but the origin of the word itself is "making whole." To make whole means healing on all levels—the mind, emotions and spirit as well as the body. As we saw in the last chapter, the use of Reiki helps to clear blockages in a person's energy field. It works holistically—healing, harmonizing and balancing the whole person—to promote better health and greater well-being. However, before we look in more depth at the ways in which Reiki can be used for healing, I want to introduce the topic of healing in a more general sense, from the way your physical body repairs itself to conventional and metaphysical approaches to healing, including looking at illness as a message from your body. You will then be able to see in later chapters how Reiki fits into the whole healing process.

THE PHYSICAL HEALING PROCESS

On a purely physical level, our bodies have an amazingly sophisticated and intelligent set of healing processes to repair and maintain themselves, from our vital organs to our bones, muscles and skin. Inside our bodies, cells are continuously lost through wear and tear and replaced by cell growth and division. At one time it was believed that a few parts of our bodies—notably, the brain and the nervous system—were unable to be repaired or replaced in this way once we reached adulthood; however, new research has shown that even these cells can replicate, given certain conditions.

During each year 98 percent of the cells in your body are replaced, so in effect you have virtually a new body each birthday. Your bone cells take about three months to regenerate your skeleton, although the calcium in the bone takes longer, about a year; your liver gradually replaces itself roughly every six weeks; your skin is renewed monthly, and your stomach lining every four days.

This constant replication and repair is what enables all physical healing to take place—without it, we would all probably bleed to death from our first childhood cut! Of course, many things can impact on your body's natural healing ability; whether you eat a healthy, balanced diet; whether you drink plenty of water so that you are not dehydrated; whether you are too tired or under a great deal of stress; your age and general state of health; and so on. For example, poor nutrition reduces healing rates and increases susceptibility to infection, which further delays healing, and studies have also proved that psychological stress has a similar delaying effect on the body's healing processes.

HEALING AS A HOLISTIC ISSUE

So from the above information you can see that healing is not something that happens "out there," something that someone else "does" to you. There is really only one "healer" of your body, and that is *you*, because your body possesses the mechanisms to heal itself, so all anyone else can do—whether that person is a doctor, a nurse, a complementary therapist or a Reiki "healer"—is to kick-start that natural process in some way, whether by conventional or alternative means.

Of course, your body copes every day with lots of potential hazards. For example, if it is invaded by a virus, such as the common cold, your immune system is mobilized, and all those rather unpleasant symptoms you experience, such as a high temperature and a runny nose, are actually the effects of your body fighting off the infection, rather than effects from the virus itself. Indeed, taking medication to lower your temperature when you have a simple cold could be undoing much of your body's good work, because the virus is being killed off by the rise in temperature (although of course there are some circumstances when it is essential to bring body temperature down if it gets dangerously high—for example, in small children).

So if your body is so good at healing itself, why are there times when it is not completely well? Why do people continue to suffer from chronic or incurable illnesses? The reason is because healing—and health—are holistic issues, not simply physical ones.

As an example, your body produces precancerous (altered) cells every day, but almost all the time your immune system detects and destroys them. However, if your immune system is not operating as effectively as usual, then it is possible that not all of them will be destroyed.

There are a number of possible reasons for this: perhaps your body is already struggling to fight off another major infection, or your immune system has been seriously affected by some stressful event such as a close bereavement (or even a happy but nevertheless stressful event like a wedding), or because your body does not have the right nutritional balance to work at optimum strength. Any of these causes, and there are many other possibilities, can be at the root of the growth of cancerous cells in an otherwise healthy body.

In many cases even if this happens, providing the immune system can return to normal working capacity fairly quickly it will tackle any early cancerous growth and destroy it, and you will be none the wiser. If the cancer develops, of course, there are various conventional medical interventions that can help: surgery, chemotherapy, radiation treatment. But you have probably also heard of people who have gone on to develop mature cancerous growths, yet who have managed to mobilize their own body to destroy the cancer, sometimes with astonishing speed, even without medical intervention.

These people always have a very positive attitude and an overwhelming determination to "get better," as well as having supportive people around them to help them to release emotional blockages and gain insight into the reasons for their illness. Also, they have generally a variety of techniques such as Reiki or spiritual healing, or other complementary therapies, to help them to activate their own healing ability, because the causes of any serious illness are likely to be complex and multileveled.

THE HEALING/CURING DICHOTOMY

This brings us to the relationship between healing and curing. Let us start by unraveling some common misconceptions. Many people use the words "healing" and "curing" interchangeably, yet they don't necessarily mean the same thing. *Curing* means to eradicate an illness or disease completely, whereas *healing* can occur on many different levels:

1. Healing on the **physical** level: this might mean eradicating an illness completely, or it could simply mean limiting or alleviating the symptoms for a time.

2. Healing on the **emotional** level: this could allow you to calm any fears and to reach an acceptance of the effects of the illness.

3. Healing on the **mental** (psychological) level: this could enable you to think differently about your illness, perhaps bringing to your attention the lessons your illness is trying to teach you, and promoting understanding of the causative issues.

4. Healing on the **spiritual** level: this could enable you to develop a more loving and forgiving relationship with yourself, or perhaps even to make a peaceful transition into death.

Let's take one graphic example to demonstrate the difference between healing and curing. In the case of someone who develops gangrene in the lower part of their leg, it may be necessary to amputate the leg below the knee in order to *cure* the illness. Hopefully, if the disease has been caught in time, the gangrene will indeed be eradicated, and in practical terms the body's normal repair and replication processes will heal the wound caused by the operation.

However, an amputation certainly does not *heal* the person, because such an operation has an enormous psychological, emotional and even spiritual impact upon the person. It can have a broad range of effects, from the way the person views themselves and how easy or how difficult it is for them to accept their new body image; to the person's relationships with other people—whether they still feel loved, or attractive, or whether they expect (or receive) rejection from others because of their disabling condition. It impacts also on the way they live their lives on an everyday level, coping with the challenges to mobility or dexterity that the loss of a limb can cause; their beliefs about their future aims, ambitions and potential, and possibly even whether they believe life is worth living anymore.

Healing is therefore a very personal thing, but many people still seem to think of it as being healing at a physical level, whereas the reality is much wider. Even medical science is at last coming around to an understanding that healing is not simply a collection of physical processes; it involves the whole person—body, mind, emotions and spirit.

A HOLISTIC AND METAPHYSICAL VIEW OF HEALING

There are three possible ways of thinking about health and healing:

1. The biomedical model

Looking at health and healing from a purely physical perspective has been the predominant Western view for several hundred years—the biomedical model of health and health care. This is sometimes referred to as allopathic or conventional medicine, and it regards the physical body as a machine or a complex set of systems and chemicals; illnesses or diseases are therefore simply malfunctions, evidence of a physical breakdown that needs to be "fixed" by an "expert."

The methods used for this are of course physical: chemicals in the form of pills, injections or sprays; minor or major surgery; radiation treatment; physical manipulation; and other similar treatments that concentrate solely on the physical symptoms and give little or no credence to anything other than physical causes. In this way, the people who are ill are often viewed, not as people, but as a diagnosis, so they are described as an "asthmatic" or a "diabetic," for example.

From this viewpoint, people are seen as helpless victims—of bacteria or viruses, of faulty genes, or simply as victims of bad luck or adverse circumstances—and a person is not treated as a whole because the body is seen as a separate entity, not connected to or influenced by the mind and emotions.

2. The holistic model

Holistic is really "wholistic," meaning that the whole person is treated, so the physical body is not viewed or treated separately, but is seen as a *part* of the whole person, with the other aspects—mind, emotions, spirit, and even environment and lifestyle—being equally important.

The holistic model does not just concentrate on the symptoms of an illness or disease; it begins to look for causes. It assumes that although some physical causation is obviously a factor in illness, such as a virus or being genetically predisposed to a disease, there are also other issues to consider.

A person's state of mind, level of emotional stability, living conditions or stress at work could all be a part of his or her health crisis. For example, it is now accepted that high stress levels, such as those experienced by people facing layoffs at work or going through a divorce, deplete the immune system, leaving those affected more vulnerable to viruses or infections.

From the holistic viewpoint, unless the underlying causes of illness or disease are healed, the person will soon become ill again. The symptoms may go away temporarily, but then they will reemerge, often as something even more serious. This is the general viewpoint of complementary and alternative medicine. However, more people, including many doctors and nurses, are becoming sympathetic toward this view of health.

Patients are encouraged to look at their lives and lifestyles to see where improvements can be made, and may be persuaded to look toward complementary and alternative therapies to help them with their health problems, either by encouraging relaxation and a greater sense of harmony and balance or to help to accelerate their healing processes.

Some therapies, such as osteopathy, chiropractic, acupuncture and homeopathy, are already officially recognized as being effective—and cost-effective—alternatives to conventional medical practices, and others are becoming well respected for their proven beneficial effects, such as aromatherapy, reflexology and healing (spiritual healing and Reiki).

3. The metaphysical model

Using the metaphysical approach, everything is seen as energy, and all energy is interconnected; as we have seen, science in the form of quantum physics upholds this view. The computer on which I'm writing this book, the chair I'm sitting in, the plant on the window ledge, my own physical body and even the air that surrounds me are all energy or light, vibrating at different rates. Some are vibrating relatively slowly, which makes them dense and heavy enough to be seen and felt as physical objects, and others are vibrating very quickly, which makes them finer and lighter, like the air, for example.

From this perspective everything that we call physical or real is seen as the product of creative consciousness. Creative consciousness is described as God/dess, or the Source, The Creator, or All That Is, or even as the Universe, and since everything is connected that means that each of us, every individual, is also a part of that consciousness.

This viewpoint is very empowering but also very challenging, because it sees each of us as cocreators with God/dess, actively creating our own reality, using our consciousness or thought processes to attract events, situations or people into our lives. The metaphysical view is that everything that happens to us, everything we experience, has meaning and purpose, so there is no such thing as luck (good or bad) or coincidence, and we are not helpless victims of random events, but powerful creators of our lives, using the circumstances we create to help us to develop and grow as people—and as souls. We are spirit having a human experience, not humans having a spiritual experience.

The world we collectively create—this planet Earth—reflects the mass consciousness, the overriding beliefs, concepts, attitudes, fears and desires of the majority of people. The world we individually create—what we think, say, do, experience, whom we meet and relate to, where we live and so on—reflects our personal beliefs, concepts, attitudes, fears and desires. From this perspective there are two phrases that probably sum things up: "what you resist, persists" and "you get out what you put in."

What these both mean in slightly different ways is that what you concentrate on, you get. Therefore, if you are constantly thinking and talking negatively about something you do not want or do not like, you will constantly be re-creating it because you are still putting your conscious energy into it (that is, resisting it)—so of course it will not go away. Nothing will change until you "change your mind."

Similarly, if you put out lots of positive thoughts, words and actions, your consciousness, or conscious energy, will start to create whatever you concentrate on, so more and more good things will begin to happen. Clearly this means that your thoughts and speech are very important, because negative conscious energy attracts and manifests negative things, while positive conscious energy attracts and manifests positive things.

I know these are quite mind-blowing concepts, and some people find them very frightening, because it turns the responsibility for our lives well and truly over to us. No one else is responsible. No one else is to blame. And equally no one else deserves the credit. Not even God/dess. Pretty scary stuff! But once you get used to the idea, this viewpoint is incredibly empowering, because it puts you in the driver's seat of your life, gives you the power to change, to become who you really want to be and to live the life you really want to live.

CONSCIOUSNESS

This metaphysical approach assumes that each person's consciousness is made up of three parts:

1. The **Super-conscious**, or **Higher Self**, which is that part of us that we might call our **soul** or **spirit**; our true self, which is fully connected to the God/dess Consciousness and which has full knowledge of our life purpose and the lessons and experiences we have chosen for this life. It is that very wise part of ourselves that is totally loving and supportive, and always working with us for our greatest and highest good by subtly guiding us and

providing us with intuition and deep insight, whether we choose to acknowledge and act on this wisdom or ignore it.

2. The **Conscious Self**, sometimes referred to as the **ego**, is who we think we are, in other words, our thinking, speaking, acting self, our personality, our beliefs, attitudes, concepts, likes, dislikes and so on—everything that makes us recognizable as ourselves. The Conscious Self is not necessarily aware of the helpful insights provided by either the Higher Self or the Subconscious Self, but can operate independently until such time as the person is ready to begin to discover more about themselves, developing and growing personally and spiritually so that they become more "in tune" with the other aspects of their consciousness.

3. The **Subconscious**, which works with the Higher Self to provide intuition and insight to the Conscious Self through dreams, visualizations, instinctive "feelings" or "gut reactions" and other aspects of "**body wisdom**."

BODY WISDOM

Our physical body has its own conscious energy system, or body wisdom, which is always working for our greatest and highest good. Because of this it tries to tell us when something is going wrong, either with our thinking or in our lives generally. Its messages take the form of symptoms, illness or disease, so when we have a headache, catch a cold or flu, have a toothache or become more seriously ill, our body is trying to tell us something, trying to get us to understand the signal and do something about it. But that is the difficulty, because we don't always understand this kind of "body language," and some people are completely unaware of it, so its significance is lost.

Most people react to illness or disease by trying to get rid of the symptoms as quickly as possible, usually by seeking medical advice or intervention. A recent advertisement on television caught my attention, because it was extolling the virtues of a popular analgesic as something "for people who don't have time to have headaches."

I found this quite alarming, because while there is nothing wrong with seeking relief for symptoms, if you really want your body to be healed, you also need to understand the illness at the causative level; if you have constant headaches, "masking" them with medication and carrying on as if nothing was wrong is not a long-term solution. You are not listening to what your body is trying to tell you, so although the symptoms might abate briefly they will return because you are not taking your body's advice and acting upon it.

Your first priority is to ask yourself "*Why* am I ill?" Because from the metaphysical perspective, illness or disease is created by the body—albeit as a helpful message—and since the body is simply a part of our consciousness, this means that we actually create our own ill health. Again, this may be a very challenging concept, but as I pointed out earlier, the metaphysical viewpoint is really very empowering, because if we have the power to create ill health, then we also have the power to create good health.

However, this is definitely *not* a "blame theory." Although you may ultimately be responsible at a deep spiritual level for having created an illness, this is not being done at a conscious level so there is no blame attached, and therefore you should not harshly judge yourself—or anyone else—for being ill.

You don't suddenly wake up one morning and say "Oh, I think I'll break my leg/slip a disc/sprain my ankle today; that'll stop me from rushing around doing too much and I can have a good rest and some time to think about my direction in life!" From a human perspective that would be utter madness. But from a Soul/Higher Self/Subconscious Self level the pain of the broken leg or slipped disc or sprained ankle is simply an experience on your journey through this physical life, and it does what it is supposed to do. It stops you in your tracks, i.e., it stops you from making further progress down the wrong path.

If you heed the messages, all well and good, and you can heal and move on, but if you don't then they will lead to different life experiences, although from the soul perspective even that is still okay. All experience—good, bad or indifferent—is good experience for the growth and development of the soul, but not necessarily pleasant for a human being living through it.

I appreciate that these metaphysical theories can be very difficult to come to terms with if you have not heard them before, and they may well challenge your belief system or your concept of how the world works, and of course you are free to take them on board or ignore them—the choice is yours. But if reading about them has sparked at least an interest in finding out more, there are some recommended books in the Resources section, which you might find useful.

To summarize the metaphysical viewpoint: every illness or disease, accident or injury has a message for you, and the more serious the illness or injury, the more serious and urgent the message. Nothing is accidental or coincidental. Every experience is useful and valid and contains some valuable information for you, even some of the minor things—such as cutting your finger with a knife while chopping vegetables. Why were you distracted? What were you thinking about at the time? What are you feeling "sore" about?

UNDERSTANDING YOUR BODY'S "LANGUAGE"

Your body sends you messages every day: to highlight that something is not right in your life; to nudge you into noticing that you are going in the wrong direction; or to bring to your attention the fact that there are lessons to be learned that you are ignoring. The trouble is, we are not speaking the same language, especially if we think every "accident" is accidental, every pain is just something to be got rid of and every illness is just an inconvenience and something to be suffered until it is over.

If you are frequently unwell, could the underlying reason (or "dis-ease") be that you are unhappy or too stressed at work, but the only way you will give yourself permission to take time off is to be ill? Is being sick perhaps a way of getting more attention or affectionate responses from your family or partner? Do you "need" an illness to slow you down because you have reached a stage in your spiritual life when you need time alone for inner reflection?

These are just a few examples of the possible messages offered by the body for you to examine, learn from and then take action, making the necessary changes in your life to bring about harmony and good health. Of course, there is not room in this book to give anything other than a very short outline of some suggested metaphysical causes of illness and disease, so I have recommended some books in the Resources section that deal with this issue if you want to explore it further.

The list below shows just a few of the possible relationships between parts of the body or specific illnesses and facets of our inner selves, as a very rough guide. This list is only a brief example of a complex issue and is not intended to be regarded as the "truth" in every case.

See if they "feel" right to you; they are generalizations and each case is individual, so you may need to explore the issue in more depth. In the meantime, however, it may sound simplistic to say that if you have a sore throat you may be experiencing problems expressing yourself, but just be prepared to look at that, honestly, to see if it has any relevance for you. If not, that is fine, but please remember that most of us are very good at hiding our motivations from ourselves, so probing our deeper reasoning can be an uncomfortable and disturbing experience. Therefore even if at first you want to deny it outright, it could be worth having another look.

Causative Issues Linked with Body Parts

Left side of body Represents our feminine side and our inner journey, as well as creativity, imagination, and spiritual and psychic issues.

Right side of body Represents our masculine side and our outer journey, as well as money or job issues, or other practical, physical and material concerns.

Eyes Show how we "see" the world. What are you not prepared to see? Are you looking at things from an unhelpful perspective?

Ears What is it you are unwilling to hear? Are you avoiding listening to your inner guidance?

Throat Communication issues. Have you swallowed your anger and hurt? Are you expressing your feelings? Are you telling the truth?

Shoulders Are you carrying too many burdens? Do you always put yourself last in your list of priorities? Is your life too stressful?

Arms Who or what are you holding on to? Are you afraid to let go? Who or what would you like to embrace?

Hands Associated with giving (right hand) and receiving (left hand), and the details of life. What issues or situation can you not handle?

Back Associated with stored anger and resentment, feeling unsupported, and trying to be perfect, as well as money issues and indefinable fears.

Chest (heart/lungs) Relationship issues, self-esteem and feelings of worthlessness, suppressed emotions, feeling smothered or controlled by others.

Legs Associated with progress through life, fear of change, fear of the future, and family or parental issues. Who/what is holding you back?

Knees Linked with stubbornness, inflexibility and indecision. What decision are you afraid to make? Are you being obstinate over something?

Ankles Do you need to change direction? Is your life unbalanced?

Feet Associated with security and survival, reaching our goals or completing tasks, fear of taking the next step and being "grounded."

USING ENERGY FOR HEALING

Everyone is born with an ability to heal, because we all have our own supply of life-force energy, or *Ki*, and this can act as a healing energy if we wish.

When we cuddle a child to comfort it when it is hurt, we use our own supply of *Ki* to soothe and heal. When we spend hours talking supportively to a friend who is going through a tough time, we often feel quite drained afterward because we have been "donating" our own supply of *Ki* to help in our friend's healing process. But if we constantly give our life force away to heal other people our supply can become too depleted, and then we can gradually find ourselves becoming listless, depressed or ill.

This can also happen if we come into contact with people who are quite unconsciously "energy drains," sometimes called "energy vampires." That may sound alarming, but you might have experienced something like that—always feeling exceptionally tired when you are with a particular person, or perhaps always being very irritated or anxious around someone, even though there does not appear to be any cause.

Fortunately this type of energy draining is usually quite a rare occurrence, and the person who is sucking your energy is almost always unaware of it. However, they may be ill or just have an energy field with an unnaturally low vibration that automatically attracts higher vibrations.

SPIRITUAL HEALING

Hands-on healing has been used for thousands of years in virtually every religion, culture and society. Some healers use their own life-force energy to heal others, but they can easily become exhausted if they use too much, because the body needs sufficient time to replenish its energy supply. Other spiritual healers work by being a focus for the energies supplied by "unseen friends" or spirit guides (people in the spiritual realm who have agreed to help humanity in this way) and they place their hands to direct energy wherever their guides tell them it is needed.

However, some spiritual healers are able to draw healing energy into themselves from the Source, which then flows into the person they are healing. This method is similar to using Reiki, but I have had many spiritual healers attending my Reiki workshops, and they have all reported that the Reiki energy feels quite different to them. It seems to flow instantaneously, unlike the other healing energies they work with, which tend to build up more slowly.

This would seem to confirm that Reiki, as a unique strand of healing energy, has its own vibrational frequency; although I personally believe all healing energies come from the same source, but they may have different ways of working and different vibrations. Indeed, there is a 5,000-year-old text called *The Yellow Emperor's Classic of Internal Medicine* in the Chinese healing tradition, which states that there are 32 different kinds of *Chi* (*Ki*).

REIKI AS A TOOL FOR HEALING

It can therefore be a great advantage to work with Reiki as a healing tool because you can channel Reiki into your energy body and out through your hands. Then when you place your hands either on yourself or on another person who needs healing, the Reiki will flow without depleting your own personal reserves of life-force energy in any way. Also, because Reiki is guided by a Higher Intelligence it works holistically, so its effects are not limited to the physical body but also affect the mind, emotions and spirit, healing, harmonizing and balancing the whole, as in the following:

Physical Reiki supports and accelerates the body's own natural ability to heal itself, helping to alleviate pain and relieve other symptoms while cleansing the body of poisons and toxins. Reiki balances and harmonizes the whole energy body, promoting a sense of wholeness, a state of positive wellness and an overall feeling of well-being. It also works with a person's physical consciousness, or body wisdom, to help them develop a greater awareness of the body's real needs—for example, the right nutrition, exercise and sleep pattern.

Mental Reiki flows into all levels of a person's thinking processes, allowing them to let go of negative thoughts, concepts and attitudes, and to replace them with positivity, peace and serenity. This leads to a state of deep relaxation, with the consequent release of stress and tension. Reiki works with the energy field, especially the brow chakra (Third Eye) to enhance intuitive abilities, and it also works with all levels of a person's consciousness to encourage them to pursue their personal potential through greater insight and self-awareness.

Emotional Reiki flows into all levels of a person's emotional energy—those of which they are aware, and those they keep hidden—to encourage them to examine their emotional responses to people and situations, allowing them to let go of negative emotions such as anger or jealousy, and promoting the qualities of loving, caring, sharing, trusting and goodwill. It can also help people to channel emotional energy into creativity.

Spiritual Reiki flows into a person's whole energy body, soul and spirit, to help them to accept and love their whole self. It fosters a nonjudgmental approach to humankind, allowing them to accept every person as a soul energy on its own spiritual path, not just as a human being with all the attendant failings and frailties. It promotes the qualities of love, compassion, understanding and acceptance, and encourages a person on their personal path toward spiritual development and connectedness with the Divine.

THE NEED FOR A CHANGE IN CONSCIOUSNESS

Whether we take a conventional or a metaphysical view, any illness, pain or disease is a signal from the body to indicate that something is wrong. From the conventional viewpoint the indications are fairly basic. If we have a pain in the stomach area then a doctor will look for physical reasons, such as an ulcer, a viral infection or maybe even a grumbling appendix, and will prescribe appropriate treatment, which could range from antibiotics to surgery.

From the metaphysical point of view, the message is seen at the causative level, so a stomach pain might indicate that there is something happening in your life that you are, literally, finding "hard to stomach." Reiki usually alleviates such physical symptoms quite quickly, but because it also works at the causative level, it will help raise to the surface the issues that are at the root of the phys-ical problem.

Perhaps what you cannot "stomach" is the way you are being treated by your boss or colleagues at work, but once the stomach-ache goes away you go back to work and carry on as normal. In this case, the *cause* has not been removed even though the symptom has been relieved. Soon the tension returns and the stomachache comes back or is replaced by some other, often more serious, symptom of stress. What is needed is a *change of consciousness*: a realization that something must be done about the situation at work.

The problem needs to be tackled in a proactive way. This might mean being assertive and telling your work colleagues that you don't find their attitude acceptable, or talking to your boss about your dissatisfaction. It may even mean you really need to look for another job that you would find more enjoyable and perhaps better suited to your skills and talents, because sometimes illness can be a "wake-up call" to show us that we are not on the right track.

The main theme here is being involved in your own healing, taking responsibility for your own health and well-being. One of the best and easiest ways of helping you to do this is by learning how to use Reiki, so that you can be an active participant in your own self-healing, and that's what we deal with in the next chapter.

Chapter 4

Training in Reiki

People have lots of different reasons for attending their first Reiki course, but for many it is the desire to help others that finally motivates them to sign up for a workshop. Most of us know someone—a family member or friend—who could do with a little help with an illness or other aspects of their health, and it is natural to want to do something positive for the people we care about. Others have a wish to help themselves to get over a health problem, and have heard that with Reiki you can help yourself. Some people, however, simply want Reiki to help them to relax, or cope with frenetic, stressful lives, while others want to add it to the range of therapies they already offer to clients.

Whatever the motivation, the most frequently quoted reason seems to be that "it just felt right." People progress, personally and spiritually, through all the experiences life gives them, and it seems that when the time is right Reiki finds you, rather than you finding Reiki. It will begin to turn up in your life in some way—you will read an article in a magazine, overhear a conversation in a café, find that your best friend's just completed a course, or a book just catches your eye in your local bookstore. You may never have heard of it before, or you might have been thinking about it for some time, but there it is—Reiki.

As I explained in Chapter 2, all energy is connected, and when your Higher Self feels that Reiki is an appropriate next step for you, to help you grow both personally and spiritually, it sends out a signal, and Reiki, being guided by a Higher Intelligence, picks up the signal and finds you. From then on, it is likely to keep turning up until you get the message.

How Do People Acquire the Ability to Use Reiki?

Reiki is the simplest and easiest holistic healing method available to us, so anyone can learn to use it, whatever their age or gender, religion or origin. No specific prior knowledge or experience is required; you need only a desire to learn, a willingness to let this healing energy flow through you, and some spare time to attend a short course.

However, Reiki cannot be "learned" in any of the ways with which we in the West are familiar. You cannot acquire the ability to channel Reiki by reading a book, or attending a lecture, or watching a television program or video; although you can learn how to *use* Reiki in those ways—for example, where to place your hands when carrying out a Reiki treatment.

Reiki does not actually require any learning, in the traditional sense, because it is not knowledge-based; it is experience-based. You have to take part in a special ceremony of spiritual empowerment, usually called an attunement or initiation, where you become initiated into the Reiki energy by a qualified Reiki Master who has been taught how to carry out that process, so that you become a Reiki channel, able to draw Reiki into yourself whenever and wherever you wish to.

Becoming a Reiki Channel

The spiritual empowerment "attunes" your energy body to the particular vibrational frequencies of the Reiki energy, meaning it brings your energies and the Reiki energies into harmony with one another, so that the Reiki can flow easily into and around your energy field. This process also creates, or reactivates, a permanent spiritual channel (a type of conduit in the energy body to carry spiritual energy) within your energy field, through which Reiki (and only Reiki) can flow into your crown chakra, and through your brow, throat and heart chakras to your arms and then down to the center of each palm, and out (see illustration, page 30).

This channel is not visible (except perhaps to people with exceptional psychic gifts), but I usually describe it as an energy equivalent of a fiber-optic tube. Just as light can flow down a fiber-optic tube and be seen shining out the other end, so Reiki flows down this channel in your energy body until it flows out your hands.

"Channeling" healing energy is similar to "channeling" other forms of spiritual energy, which is something that has been a part of many spiritual traditions throughout history. It is a word that can also encompass forms of mediumship, communicating with spirit guides (human spirits who have lived before and whose work is now to help humans to follow their own spiritual path), "speaking in tongues" and other mystical experiences. Some Reiki Masters claim to have "channeled" additional symbols, or new methods of attunement, or specific hand positions to enhance their healing, and other people speak of "channeling" information from highly evolved spiritual guides.

What this means in real terms is that they have received insight and inspiration they believe to be from a source outside of themselves, or possibly from their Souls/Higher Selves, which may take place during meditation or visualization, during a creative activity or simply when walking in natural surroundings. For some of these people this can produce a very profound spiritual experience of a psychic nature, while for others it seems more like a perfectly normal part of everyday life, like waking up from a powerful and enlightening dream. Channeling Reiki, on the other hand, is simple, easy and automatic once you have been attuned to its energetic vibration; it requires no rituals or complicated processes and it feels perfectly natural.

THE LEVELS OF TRAINING

There are normally three levels of training, although sometimes you may encounter Reiki Masters who split the training into four, five or even seven parts. The levels are usually described as Reiki 1, 2 and 3 or Reiki I, II and III or often as Reiki First, Second and

Third Degrees—but this does not refer to (or confer) any academic level or qualification.

THE ATTUNEMENT/INITIATION PROCESS

"Attune" means to bring into harmony, and the process of being "attuned" to the energetic frequency of Reiki is how you are "initiated" into Reiki, how you become a "channel" for Reiki. The attunement process makes Reiki unique, and is the reason why the ability to heal can be developed so quickly, yet so permanently. It is a sacred ceremony of spiritual empowerment, and the actual process is kept secret until someone becomes a Reiki Master, when the Reiki 3 student is taught the Master Symbol and the attunement procedure for each of the three levels of Reiki.

As I have described earlier, the attunement carried out in a Reiki class is a version of the spiritual empowerment that Dr. Usui received on Mount Kurama, but gentler and less powerful than he experienced. It forms a connection among the student, the Master and the Reiki energy, and it is carried out in what I would describe as "sacred space."

When the Reiki Master "brings in" the energy in order to commence the attunement, this has the effect of altering the space around the Master and student(s), filling it with Reiki to provide a protective environment. When I am carrying out an attunement I can always feel this difference, and some students also remark upon it afterward, but on some occasions I have actually seen this take place, and the whole room seems to be bathed in violet light.

Another effect is that the Reiki Master becomes filled with Reiki in a very tangible way and, again, I always see and feel this. On several occasions I have taught Reiki in a dance studio, which had mirrors down one side, and as I carried out the attunements I looked up and saw my reflection, and was amazed to see myself surrounded by a very visible bright golden aura, spreading out to at least 2 meters (6½ ft) around and above me, and I could also see the stream of Reiki coming down into my crown chakra. Also, every time I carry out attunements I notice an incredible increase in my body heat as the Reiki fills me, and this is one reason why I limit the number of students I teach in a class, as the more students I have, the greater the amount of energy I have to carry, so the hotter I get!

What Happens in an Attunement?

Although each attunement has the same elements, each Reiki Master decides exactly how an attunement should be carried out, and sometimes this will depend on the way the Master prefers to teach. Some Masters like to teach on a one-to-one basis, so they will obviously carry out the attunement process on one individual. Other Masters teach groups of students, so they will usually gather all the students together, generally seated on chairs set out in a straight line, a circle, or a horseshoe shape. However, sometimes even if the Master teaches a group, they may prefer to perform the whole attunement on one student at a time, so any other students in the class are asked to wait in another room and take turns to receive the attunement.

Whichever way a Master prefers to operate, they will usually set out the room according to their own preferences, and often this will include having candles and incense burning and possibly a small altar with crystals and other sacred objects on it. Although none of these additions is essential, they help to highlight the special and sacred nature of the attunement.

The room will then be cleansed with Reiki, to help to create a "sacred space," and the students will be invited to take their seats. Before the attunement begins, the Master will normally explain to the student(s) what to expect and will then ask them to hold their hands in the prayer position (called *Gassho* in Japanese) with their thumbs pointing to the middle of the chest. They will then be asked to close their eyes and to keep them closed throughout the whole procedure. The attunement is normally carried out in silence, although appropriate soft background music may be played.

When the students have settled, the Master will begin by quietly "tuning in" to the Reiki vibrations before connecting with and channeling into the self sufficient Reiki energy to carry out the spiritual empowerment. The process is carried out with the Master standing initially behind the student, then in front, and ending behind the student again. At various stages during the process there may be some gentle touching on the student's head and hands, and the student may be asked to raise his or her hands above the head for a few moments, but everything is gentle, supportive and restful.

The attunement is a very special, meditative experience, and the silent contemplation with eyes closed is performed for two reasons. The first is obviously because, as a sacred and spiritual ceremony, the procedures are intended to be kept secret until such time as any individual student trains to be a Reiki Master. The second, less obvious reason is that when someone has their eyes closed, this reduces any external distractions around them, stilling the mind so that they are more easily able to stay in an appropriate meditative state, which leaves them more receptive to and aware of a mystical experience.

Being initiated into Reiki is a powerful spiritual experience, although how it is experienced will vary from person to person, as the Rei, or God-consciousness, guides the whole process, adjusting it according to the needs of each individual. After the attunements are over, students often describe the beautiful spiritual or mystical experiences they have enjoyed, such as "seeing" wonderful colors, or visions of beautiful healing places. Others report receiving personal insights or profound healing, sensing the presence of spirit guides or angelic beings or simply having a feeling of complete peace.

The attunement creates a permanent energetic channel in your energy body, through which Reiki (and only Reiki) can flow. At the end of each attunement, the Master "seals" the channel, so from then on you have your own direct connection with Reiki, and no longer need to have it channeled through the Master.

THE EFFECTS OF ATTUNEMENT TO REIKI

Attunement is only the *start* of your connection to Reiki, and over the ensuing weeks and months as you practice using it, the flow of Reiki gains strength so that within six to eight weeks after being initiated into Reiki you are experiencing the full flow of energy. Basically, the more you use it, the better it flows, and once you have received a Reiki attunement you will be able to use Reiki for the rest of your life. It does not wear off or wear out, the supply of Reiki is inexhaustible, and you can never lose the ability to channel it.

However, if for some reason you don't use Reiki for a long time, you may think it is not flowing because you don't have any sensation of it in your hands. Some people ask to be reattuned if this happens, but there really is no need, because it is still there—you just need to carry out some self-cleansing (which will be described later) and practice to bring back the full flow. However, if you choose to undertake a reattunement, it will not do any harm; it can be another pleasant experience and will also increase the amount of Reiki you can channel.

At each level of attunement (Reiki 1, 2 or 3) you become able to tap into a higher, wider channel of Reiki healing energy, and the vibrationary rate of your energy body is increased. Some people go through a shift in their awareness immediately, describing the sensation as almost like being reborn, so that they experience everything around them more intensely: colors are brighter, their sense of smell is enhanced and sounds are sharper. Others feel a buzzing or heightened sensitivity in the crown chakra for a short while or describe a sense of floating or light-headedness. All of these reactions are absolutely normal. However, experiencing very little is quite common too, and while it may be a little disappointing for some students, it definitely does *not* mean the attunement has not worked.

Because Reiki is guided by a Higher Intelligence, it therefore adjusts to suit each person, so everyone's experience of a Reiki attunement is slightly different, even though the process is identical for everyone. If someone has already been doing energy work for some time—perhaps t'ai chi, chi kung or martial arts, or they already do some form of spiritual healing—then their bodies are already tuned in to higher energetic vibrations, so they are able to absorb and channel more Reiki right from the moment they are attuned.

The same is often true of people who have done a lot of spiritual work, including deep meditation. However, if a person has never done anything in terms of energy or spiritual work they will still be able to channel Reiki, but the flow of energy they experience may be less initially. After a few weeks of practice, however, there is very little difference between the amount of Reiki flowing through the energetically or spiritually experienced and that flowing through an inexperienced person.

It is this unique attunement process that is one of the major differences between Reiki and other "hands-on healing" methods. It
is possible to learn how to channel other forms of spiritual healing,
and there are various organizations that teach it, such as the
National Federation of Spiritual Healers in the U.K., and similar
establishments in other countries. However, it can take many
months to learn and, as I explained earlier, the energy channeled
by spiritual healers is not Reiki but energy of a different vibration.

The channel that is created during the Reiki spiritual empowerment becomes active immediately, so within minutes you can
begin to draw Reiki through yourself, which can then be used either
for your own healing or to heal others. From then on, whenever you intend to use Reiki, simply thinking about it, or holding your hands out in readiness to use it, will activate it—there are
no complicated rituals to follow.

Reiki does not flow through you all the time, however. You can
put out your hand to pick up a cup of tea, for instance, and that
will not switch the Reiki on! What starts the Reiki flowing is your
intention to use it. Later, when you have been using Reiki for some
time, you may find that the Reiki "switches on" without you actively
intending it to happen, but if you have been practicing Reiki quite
a lot on yourself and on others your unspoken intention is to use
Reiki whenever it is needed. As it is Divinely guided, if there is a
person (or an animal) nearby who is really in need of it, then their
Higher Self (and animals have a form of higher consciousness too)
will know that you are a Reiki channel, and will request it. The
Reiki will just respond, because on a subconscious level you have
given permission. You have chosen to become a Reiki channel.

This process can only happen, however, because Reiki is *pulled* by
the recipient, not *pushed* by the Practitioner. Healing cannot be
forced onto anyone. However, this does not have to be a conscious
process either for the Practitioner or the recipient, because it is
controlled by the recipient's Higher Self. Therefore, the person
receiving the Reiki does not need to do anything or think about
anything in particular. It is helpful if the recipient is consciously
willing to receive the energy but even this is not strictly necessary.
Reiki will flow into animals, and they don't know what it is.

If a person's Soul/Higher Self knows they need healing, it will
draw Reiki into the person's energy body, overriding any conscious

objections. When I do public demonstrations of Reiki, I often come across people who are very skeptical and who patently don't believe Reiki can work. However, if they can be persuaded to allow me to place my hands on their shoulders to see if the Reiki will flow they are almost without exception astonished at the results, and often they are then the first to sign up to take a Reiki course.

Sensations of Reiki Flowing Through Your Hands

Another effect following a Reiki attunement is that whenever you intend it to, Reiki begins to flow out of the palms of your hands. The way in which students experience this is very varied. As I explained earlier, Reiki adjusts to suit each recipient; some people are fairly clear channels to start with, and in those instances more Reiki can flow through them; the more Reiki flows through, the more sensation you are likely to get. But people sense energy in different ways.

Some people experience the world in a very visual way, so they might see the energy as colors, getting very little physical sensation in their hands. Others experience the world kinesthetically, being much more aware of physical sensations caused by the flow of energy—they may even experience the energy as a taste or a smell, although this is less usual.

When they place their hands on themselves, or on others, to do Reiki, some people have immediate feelings in their hands of heat or gentle warmth, a cool sensation as though a breeze was blowing on them, or they sense tingling, prickling, tickling or buzzing in their hands and fingers. A few even experience these sensations going up their arms as well, and occasionally these sensations are experienced in the crown chakra, too.

Other people, however, feel nothing at all and are naturally disappointed, especially if they compare their experience with that of others who are exclaiming about all these sensations. Their natural concern is that the attunement has not worked, or they are just no good at Reiki.

This certainly is not the case. An attunement always works. It has a 100 percent success rate all of the time. It is not possible to fail a Reiki course, provided a qualified Reiki Master carries out the attunement process with you. You will be able to channel Reiki. But you will not necessarily feel anything, at least at first.

If there are lots of blockages in your energy body it might take a little longer to establish a full flow, so you may gradually begin to experience some sensations after a few weeks or months—provided you use Reiki. If you just give up straightaway you are unlikely to clear the blockages sufficiently to get the Reiki flowing fully. You have still retained the ability to channel Reiki; you just are not using it.

Rid yourself of the idea that there are people who are "no good at Reiki"; everyone who has been attuned has roughly the same potential to be a good Reiki channel, and the Reiki that flows through a brand-new Reiki First Degree student is exactly the same as the Reiki that flows through their initiating Reiki Master. It does not flow as much or as fast, but it is the quality, not the quantity, that counts. True, a few people do turn out to be outstanding at channeling Reiki—and being treated by them is fabulous, like being under a waterfall of pure healing. But that ability is rare, and I have no plausible explanation for it.

MULTIPLE ATTUNEMENTS

Some students enjoy attunements so much that they want to repeat the experience as often as possible, which is one of the reasons why some people choose to progress very quickly through Reiki 1, 2 and 3. Other people choose instead to attend several Reiki courses at the same level but with different Masters, sometimes because they are under the (mistaken) impression that they have not been attuned "properly," or that because they have not used their Reiki for months—or years—it will not work anymore, which is another mistaken belief. Some Reiki Masters are very much against this, but although I would not wish to encourage people to become "attune-ment junkies," there is nothing intrinsically wrong with having a number of attunements at the same level, as each attunement helps to widen the Reiki channel, enabling even more Reiki to flow through.

Indeed, you may remember that in Japan it is usual for Reiki students to gather together about once a month with their Master to share treatments, ask questions and receive a simple attunement/empowerment called *Rei-ju*. This is not identical to the attunement process used to initiate a person during a Reiki course, but it does increase the power and flow of the Reiki they can channel and is beneficial for their spiritual development, too.

Waiting for a reasonable time between attunements is sensible because it allows your physical body to adjust to the new, higher vibrationary rate that results from the previous attunement. This is the case whether you intend to take several attunements at the same level with the same or different Masters, and is even more important if you want to progress from Reiki 1 to Reiki 2, or from Reiki 2 to Reiki 3.

At each level of Reiki training the attunement expands your Reiki channel. This increases the amount of Reiki that can flow through you and also raises the vibrations and frequency of your energy body. I recommend a minimum of three months between Reiki First and Second Degree (most of my students choose to wait at least a year), and then a minimum of three years of active Reiki practice on yourself and others at Second Degree level before being attuned at Third Degree/Master level. This gives you time to gather practical experience of treatments, and also time to carry out self-healing, which is vital for everyone, but especially for those who want to be professional Practitioners or who wish to become Reiki Masters.

AFTER AN ATTUNEMENT

Apart from the experiences I have already described, some people find that they are very hungry during and after a Reiki course or they need much more sleep than usual. This is probably because they are not used to the higher vibrational energy flowing through them, so it is rather like getting your physical body going when you first start exercising—it is just tiring. Others, conversely, seem to have lots of extra energy—but that just demonstrates that each person has an individual experience of Reiki.

Most people do feel on a "high"—buzzing with excitement and enthusiasm—when they have finished the course, because for many an attunement is definitely a peak experience, so I recommend that when you have attended a Reiki workshop you try to slip back into normal life as gently as possible afterward. This may not be easy, as often the courses are held during a weekend and you may have to get back to work on Monday. However, if you do have the chance to take an extra day off, just allow yourself to "come down" slowly, perhaps sleeping longer and then spending the day doing gentle things like walking, reading, meditating or listening to relaxing music—and giving yourself Reiki.

After each level of attunement the vibrationary rate at which you operate is raised—the norm is 250 cps (cycles per second) but healers range from 400 to 800 cps. In order for this to happen there has to be a clearing of old physical, mental, emotional and spiritual patterns and thoughts that inhibit the growth of consciousness. One of the major effects of an attunement, therefore, is what is called the 21-day clearing process, where your whole energy body is cleansed and cleared by the Reiki. This is not a permanent effect, however, so you will need to use Reiki to cleanse your energy system quite regularly, but there are details of this in a later chapter.

21-day Clearing Process

This usually takes about three weeks—hence, the title—but can sometimes be accomplished more quickly, or take a little longer. During the first few weeks after each Reiki attunement, at whatever level, the Reiki that flowed into your physical and energy bodies so powerfully during the attunement begins to work on clearing specific parts of your auric field associated with the physical, emotional, mental and spiritual aspects of the self.

It does this through the chakras, clearing, harmonizing and balancing one chakra each day for the first week, and then the cycle repeats itself as often as necessary until the clearing work is completed, which is why it may take less than three weeks or as long as five, six or seven weeks depending upon how much clearing and balancing work is required.

The clearing begins gradually, starting at the root or base chakra on day one, and continuing to the sacral chakra on day two, the solar plexus chakra on day three and so on, right up to the crown chakra on day seven. During the clearing process you may find that facets of your life associated with each of the chakras are highlighted, perhaps through dreams or memories, or people coming back into your life to trigger certain thoughts and feelings to help you let go of them. The following points might help you to identify these areas, and they also describe what some people call the four etheric bodies—physical, emotional, mental and spiritual—within your energy field.

PHYSICAL

Two chakras are most closely associated with your physical energies. The root chakra, which is related to your basic survival instinct and feelings of security, can trigger issues about money, your home and job and your physical body. The sacral chakra relates to physical sensations and sexuality, so issues of intimacy and sex, as well as those associated with food, appetite and other sensual pleasures, can come up.

EMOTIONAL

The two chakras associated with emotional energies are the solar plexus and the heart. With the solar plexus chakra, issues to do with your feelings and beliefs about yourself might come up, such as autonomy, life purpose, willpower and self-esteem, while the heart chakra's issues link to your ability to love unconditionally and include giving and receiving, compassion for others and loving acceptance of yourself.

MENTAL

The throat and brow chakras are associated with your mental energies. The throat chakra throws up issues about communication, self-expression and your sense of deservingness. With the brow chakra, also called the third eye, issues raised might include psychic and spiritual awareness, your ability to respond to intuition or insight, and your recognition of yourself as a unique individual consciousness.

SPIRITUAL

The crown chakra is linked with your spiritual energies, and issues about knowledge and intellect, as well as your capacity to understand on a deeper, more spiritual level, may be raised, including a desire to explore aspects of mystical union with the Divine and connection with all life.

During the second and third weeks, this clearing cycle is repeated in the same way—root chakra on day one, sacral chakra on day two and so on. I usually describe this to my students as a sort of energetic "spring cleaning," where the Reiki gently flows through and breaks down the blockages in your whole energy system.

As the blocks that are preventing your progress are brought forward, the trapped and blocked energies need to be released by your energy body. Sometimes this is achieved quite easily and you may feel colder than usual, as energy while being released often has an icy feel. The intensity of the clearing and the way it is experienced depends upon each person, as everyone is unique, with their own personal life experiences, thought patterns, emotional baggage and so on.

The effects of the release of any blockages can vary from feeling more emotional or irritable than usual or having the urge to laugh or cry frequently to a sense of detachment and the need to spend more time alone. Other blocked energy may need to be released through your physical body, however, and you may experience a temporary "healing crisis," such as having a cold or sweating a lot, or even occasionally being sick or having diarrhea for a while. These are simply ways to release toxins from the body and they are perfectly natural (if a little uncomfortable), so please don't be alarmed. However, these effects don't always happen, so don't turn them into a "self-fulfilling prophecy."

The reason some people occasionally experience more severe physical reactions is usually because there are deeper blockages to release—for example, perhaps they are harboring deep resentment against someone, either consciously or subconsciously.

These intense emotional feelings have to be cleared from the energy body, and since they can be represented by almost tangible, dense energy, they need to flow into the physical body in order to be released. The easiest route is through the body's excretory system, but if the body is in any way dehydrated other more extreme routes may need to be chosen (like vomiting), because it is in the body's best interest to be rid of this toxic energy as quickly as possible. Another reason this can happen is that the person is spiritually ready to release and clear issues on a deeper level, although this may be more likely to happen after a Second Degree or Master-level attunement.

It is important to remember, however, that Reiki is Divinely guided and therefore always works for the highest good, so you can trust Reiki to know what is best for you and to do it—even if that sometimes results in some temporary discomfort.

Helping the Clearing Process

You can make the whole process as easy as possible for yourself by following these suggestions:

- Do lots of Reiki on yourself, especially a full Reiki self-treatment (see Chapter 6) of at least half an hour every day during this clearing cycle.

- Drink *lots* of water—at least six to eight glasses (approximately 2 liters/3½ pints a day). This needs to be pure water (other drinks, like tea, coffee, cordials, beer, fizzy drinks, and so on, don't count) but can be either bottled or (preferably) filtered tap water. Seltzer is okay very occasionally, but since the carbon dioxide that makes it fizzy is actually one of your body's waste products, you are accumulating more toxins. It is also best to drink the water plain, rather than adding any flavors. *Note that if you have any health problems, particularly any related to water retention, you should seek medical advice before drinking extra water.*

- Try to reduce your intake of obvious toxins such as alcohol, cigarettes or other drugs (but do *not* reduce the dosage of any drugs or medicines prescribed by your doctor).

- It is also helpful to eat very healthily at this time, concentrating on fresh foods, particularly organic vegetables and fruits, rather than prepackaged meals and other products, which often contain lots of additives and preservatives.

Over the 21 days, and for a number of weeks afterward, you will probably notice a gradual strengthening of the Reiki as you use it, as well as other changes in yourself. For this reason I often suggest to my students that they keep a journal of their "Reiki journey" for the first few weeks, where they can record what they experience during self-treatment, or during treatments of friends, family, pets or plants. They also find it a good idea to write down any vivid dreams, emotional episodes, feelings or meditations they experience, or changes they feel are taking place in themselves—and perhaps link them to the particular chakra that is being "cleared" on that day.

Part II

Activating Your Healing Channel—Reiki First Degree

Chapter 5

Reiki First Degree Training

Once you have made the decision to take a Reiki course, you need to find the Reiki Master who is right for you. Actually *find* is probably the wrong word because Reiki is a Divinely guided energy and, when the time is right, Reiki finds you, rather than the other way around. Also, it always guides you to the Master who will give you exactly what you need—because Reiki always works for your highest and greatest good. Every Master is unique and each one of them brings something of themselves to their teaching, so of course it is important that you should feel that they are someone you can like, trust and respect.

HOW TO FIND THE REIKI MASTER FOR YOU

People find their Reiki Master in all sorts of ways—by seeing a poster in a complementary health clinic, reading an advertisement in a magazine or being recommended by a friend. Let your intuition and your common sense guide you and you will not go far wrong. Some people prefer to get to know their potential Master before making a final choice, and probably the best way is to make an appointment to have at least one Reiki treatment from them, because that will also help you to know what Reiki really is.

Other Masters offer an introductory evening session where they demonstrate and talk about Reiki, often held the evening before a course, without putting you under any obligation to join the course the next day. Then you can discuss the possibility of training with them and you are always free to go away and think about it.

To help you make an informed decision there are some questions you might like to ask, such as how the Master structures the courses, what is included, whether there is time in the course for supervised practice and so on. You might also like to know how many years they have been teaching and whether they operate as a Practitioner, so that they can give practical advice and have plenty of experience to use as examples, as well as whether they host regular Reiki sharing sessions where students can get together to practice Reiki and give each other treatments. You might also want to know whether the Master has trained in additional techniques from the Japanese tradition, or if they also teach meditation or other spiritual workshops, because this could give an added depth and dimension to their teaching.

The location of the course will be another factor in your decision. It could be important to you to train with someone in your local area so that you can meet with them later to discuss any areas of concern, or you might be prepared to travel to another area to train with a particular Master and keep in touch by phone or e-mail afterward.

Some Masters travel widely, running courses at many different venues, while others work only in their own area, perhaps teaching at a local holistic center or in their own home. I usually like to teach my courses as weekend residentials in one or two centrally located venues that include overnight accommodation and meals so that students are able to travel there easily from all over the country. I find that this also allows them to take the necessary "time out" from their normal, busy lives, making the course an even more special experience.

Your choice of Reiki Master is important because the initiation process at each level of Reiki creates a very profound connection between the Reiki Master and the student. It is therefore essential that the attunement is given by someone who embodies the energy of Reiki.

In the West we tend to distrust what cannot be explained, and a sacred spiritual experience, which empowers you with Reiki for the rest of your life, would certainly fall into that category. You need to feel personally and energetically comfortable and at ease with the

Reiki Master, and to feel inspired by their example. You need to have confidence that they have both the technical knowledge of how an attunement is performed and the spiritual knowledge and experience to carry out the process mindfully, because being attuned to Reiki can be likened to opening a door to the Divine. You presumably would not open the door of your home to people you did not like or trust, and the same should be true of your relationship with your Reiki Master, whom you are inviting to open a door into your very being.

At the end of the day, the Reiki Master you find will be the right one for you. If you like practical, no-nonsense people, you will probably be attracted to train with someone similar; if you are a real go-getter who cannot bear to wait for things, you will find a Master who is willing to let you progress quickly through the levels. If you love history and tradition, you will probably choose a very traditional Reiki Master; and if you are very interested in spirituality, you will find a Master who teaches mainly from that perspective. The point is that nowadays the choices are out there.

In 1991, when I took my Reiki 1, there were very few Reiki Masters around—probably not even a dozen in the whole of the U.K.—and all of them were very traditional in their approach. I am not complaining about that because it was absolutely the right experience for me at the time. Since then there has been a great shift in the way Reiki is taught, and this has allowed an explosion in numbers, so there are now many hundreds—possibly thousands— of Reiki Masters in the U.K. and hundreds of thousands elsewhere in the world. Now there are as many different types of Reiki Master as there are different types of people, which just means that everyone can find someone who suits them, and Reiki can continue to grow and spread rapidly around the world.

PREPARING FOR A REIKI COURSE

When you have found the right Reiki Master, you are ready to book a workshop at a convenient time and place. There are some advantages to preparing yourself before taking a Reiki course. A Reiki attunement is a special, spiritual experience and as such the experience can be enhanced if you bring all of your energies—physical, emotional, mental and spiritual—into harmony and balance during the week before a course commences.

Some aspects of our lives make this more difficult, so you might like to follow the suggestions below, but of course they are optional. There are no serious disadvantages to not preparing for a Reiki course, so don't worry if you are reading this the night before attending one or if you did a course ages ago but did not do any of this. They are just about getting the most out of the more spiritual aspects of the course, plus they help to reduce the toxins in your body, which makes the clearing process after the course a bit easier. Please note that some of them involve changing your diet, which for most people is beneficial, but if you have any health problems or feel concerned in any way, seek medical advice first.

- It can be helpful to do a gentle "detox" for a few days before an attunement, eating mostly raw fresh vegetables and fruit—preferably organic—and drinking plenty of water. If you are accustomed to fasting, you might wish to start with 24 hours on a water or fruit/vegetable-juice fast.

- If that sounds a bit too drastic, then even if you are not a vegetarian you may find it helpful to cut out meat, poultry and fish for a few days before the course. They can all contain small quantities of drugs or other toxins, and their energetic vibrations could also contain negativity from the fear the animals experience during the catching, transporting and slaughtering processes. Instead, substitute lots of fresh organic fruits and vegetables, and also cut down or eliminate processed foods, which contain preservatives and additives.

- Try to drink plenty of water—the body needs about 2 liters (3½ pints) a day to operate optimally, some of which it can extract from the foods and beverages you take in, but you make your body's work much easier if you give it what it needs. *Remember to check with your doctor if you have any reason to suspect that an increased water intake could be detrimental.*

- It is best to eliminate alcohol for a few days before and during the Reiki course, and possibly for a few days afterward. Also, try to minimize your consumption of caffeine drinks such as tea, coffee and cola; other fizzy drinks; sweet or fatty foods; and chocolate.

- If you smoke, try to cut down for several days beforehand and smoke as little as possible during and immediately after the course. If you take any drugs, try to limit or eliminate your consumption of them for as long as possible before, during and after the course—*but do not cut out or reduce the dosage of any drugs or medicines prescribed for you by your doctor*.

- Try to reduce or eliminate altogether any time you spend in any activities or situations that carry negative energy, such as watching the television news, or violent or fear-inducing programs or films; reading newspapers or books containing violence or horror; listening to loud music; being with people who have very negative views, or being in places that make you feel uncomfortable.

- Take some time out for yourself to spend quietly in contemplation or meditation or walking in a park or the countryside, or listening to classical or "New Age" music, as these are useful activities to "destress" you so that you will be more in tune with the nature of the course.

All of the above suggestions can contribute to a healthier long-term lifestyle too, and you may find that after the Reiki course you will want to live more healthily. For example, some people find it much easier to give up smoking after being attuned to Reiki, and even more find that healthy eating is an attractive option, because the Reiki makes them more aware of the toxic load they may have habitually taken into their bodies.

WHAT TO EXPECT IN A REIKI FIRST DEGREE COURSE

Courses (sometimes called classes, workshops or seminars) are usually relaxed and informal, and are often held at weekends, or on consecutive evenings during the week to allow more people an opportunity to attend. In the West, until the mid-1990s, the First

Degree was traditionally taught over four sessions—for two or four days, or four evenings—especially when taught by members of the Reiki Alliance. This gave a minimum of 12 hours of teaching and included four separate attunements, allowing the Reiki energy to build up slowly over the four sessions, plus a comprehensive explanation of the Usui Reiki Healing System, as Mrs. Takata had taught it.

This consisted of the story of how Reiki was discovered by Dr. Usui, plus full training in the hand positions on the head and body for treating yourself and other people, and advice on how to use Reiki in cases of injuries or accidents, as well as using it with animals and plants. Time would be allowed for practicing treatments on yourself and with other students, and for asking questions and sharing experiences, but it was taught as an oral tradition, so no notes were taken or handouts given to students.

Some Masters, myself included, still prefer to teach Reiki in this way, although most of us now provide a set of class notes or even a comprehensive manual, and include more up-to-date information about Dr. Usui and his discovery of Reiki.

Here is an example of how a traditional Reiki First Degree course in the West is normally organized. It includes the introductory session, which many Masters offer, so that anyone interested can find out more about Reiki. There may be minor variations, but it is fairly typical:

Friday

A typical evening introductory meeting covers what Reiki is, how it was discovered, what it can be used for and an explanation of the three levels of training. There is also a demonstration, giving each person the opportunity to experience receiving Reiki for a few minutes, and a question-and-answer session. (I also include a practical look at the human energy body, including using dowsing rods to detect the layers of the aura, plus sensing with the hands and seeing the human aura and how this relates to Reiki, but not all Masters do this.)

Saturday

The first day of the course usually starts with introductions so that people can begin to feel comfortable with one another. The rest of the day includes more information about what Reiki is, how it works, and some of the ways in which it can be used. Students are told what an attunement is and then the first of four attunements is given, usually toward the end of the morning, and a second in the afternoon. (Some Masters lead a short meditation before each attunement.) A discussion of the Reiki Principles follows and the importance of self-treatment with Reiki is also discussed, demonstrated and practiced. Sometimes there is time for a further practical session where students begin using Reiki on each other.

Sunday

The second day includes the other two attunements, the third being given quite early in the morning session and the fourth just after lunch. (It is preferable to have at least four hours between the attunements.) There is an explanation and demonstration of the hand positions to give a full Reiki treatment and then students are split up into pairs to practice on each other. Afterward there is a discussion of some creative ways of using Reiki, including dealing with emergencies and healing animals and plants, as well as a question-and-answer session and presentation of Reiki First Degree certificates.

Over the past ten years many independent Masters have chosen to reduce the teaching time to one day or two evenings or even half a day or one evening. These shorter workshops usually entail a single, nontraditional integrated attunement that "delivers" the energy all at once. These classes don't often include any practice time for treatments, although usually some notes are given to participating students. Occasionally a Master offers just an attunement to Reiki without any teaching backup. Very short courses, or just going through an attunement process, can lead to some confusion, and students who have no knowledge or experience of how to use Reiki for treatments or other purposes seem to have very little confidence in their ability to channel Reiki and often abandon the idea, assuming that it does not work.

Sometimes, however, Reiki courses include lots of "extras," some of which can be very beneficial, such as learning about energy, auras and chakras, being shown additional hand positions for specific ailments, or relaxation techniques using Reiki with meditation and visualization. Other extras can be a bit confusing, such as

using crystals or color healing, because although they are interesting they don't necessarily relate to Reiki.

Another variation is in class size. Many Reiki Masters teach
groups of students at the same time, some preferring small groups
of between 4 and 6 people; others have groups of up to 12 or 14.
Some have much larger gatherings of between 20 and 30, and a few
have as many as 80 students in a class. Other Masters prefer to
work on a one-to-one basis or with only two students at a time. You
need to work out for yourself what you would prefer, as there are
advantages and disadvantages to each.

Being taught individually gives you lots of time to ask questions,
but can be quite intense and there is no one else to practice on
other than the Reiki Master, which might make some students
nervous in case they make a "mistake." Being in a pair has similar
results although you have each other to practice on, but it is quite
important that you like each other if you are going to work together so closely.

Small or medium-sized groups give you a chance to practice on
a number of people, rather than just one, and you have the opportunity of meeting other like-minded people and making friends,
and possibly getting together later to practice Reiki with each other.
These groups also provide the likelihood that someone else might
ask the questions you would like to have asked, but were too shy!
Very large groups of thirty or more people obviously allow for less
individual attention from the Reiki Master, but they do give you the
advantage of anonymity if you like to get lost in a crowd.

I personally prefer to work with groups of about ten students,
as this provides enough people to form a friendly, supportive
group but does not overwhelm anyone and gives me time to take
a personal interest in each person. It also usually guarantees a
wide variety of personalities and interests, which leads to lively discussion and lots of questions, providing a healthy learning environment.

WHEN NOT TO TAKE A COURSE

There are very few times when it might be inadvisable to attend a
Reiki course, but there are some contraindications. If a person is

suffering from depression or other psychological disorders, such as schizophrenia, while in the long term it would probably be beneficial for them to be able to do Reiki on themselves, in the short term receiving a Reiki attunement could potentially intensify their symptoms.

I would therefore advise them to consider having plenty of Reiki treatments first, until their condition became more stable, and I would also recommend that they seek medical advice, suggesting that they give their doctor permission to telephone the Reiki Master for further information. (Few doctors know much about Reiki, so just asking them if it is okay is not very helpful.) Some Reiki Masters are also qualified doctors, so this would seem to be the ideal compromise, as they would be able to deal with any medical complications that arose.

Some other medical conditions also require caution. People with very high blood pressure or epilepsy or those fitted with pacemakers are probably best obtaining medical advice in the same way, although I have never experienced any problems with such people in my classes. However, because there is a slight risk that their symptoms could be intensified, if only briefly, it is probably best to err on the side of caution. The same applies to people who have recently had major surgery or who are recovering from a serious illness.

For all of these cases I would recommend Reiki treatments first, until they are confident that their health has improved. As I have said, the risks are very small, and because I am confident that Reiki always works for the highest and greatest good perhaps there are no real risks at all. Still, being a Reiki Master is a big enough responsibility without having to deal with medical complications, so it is better to be safe than sorry.

Some people become concerned about whether an attunement will affect the high levels of medication they are on, because of the cleansing of toxins that the Reiki carries out immediately afterward. Again, I have not encountered any problems in this area, and because Reiki works for the highest and greatest good, I don't believe it would ever rid the body of substances that were actually helping the person.

After using Reiki on themselves for several weeks or months, some people do find that they are able to reduce their levels of medication. However, please never do this without seeking medical advice and perhaps working with your doctor and increasing the frequency of medical checks you receive regularly, such as blood tests, to ensure that everything is proceeding smoothly.

Another condition I often get asked about is pregnancy. I have attuned a number of pregnant women, and there have never been any ill effects—other than some slight discomfort because the babies they were carrying became very lively during the attunement process. Actually, there are very real benefits for an expectant mother to be able to use Reiki, because she can use it on herself and her baby before the birth to help ease aches and pains and encourage restfulness and to promote both pain relief and relaxation during the birth. After the birth, of course, Reiki can be used to accelerate the mother's healing and to relax the baby and help both to sleep well.

It is probably only on ethical grounds that I would advise caution here, because I cannot be sure whether when the mother becomes attuned to Reiki the baby might also become attuned—although I suspect not—and the baby has no choice. One way in which this can be clarified is by the mother taking some time to "tune in" to her own and her baby's Higher Selves to ask permission; if it feels fine, then go ahead.

AFTER THE COURSE

It is a good idea to treat yourself gently for a day or two after the course, as you may find that you feel more emotional or vulnerable than usual or that your temper gets frayed more easily, but these effects generally only last for a short time. If you have to go straight back to work afterward then try to give yourself some quiet time after work and maybe go to bed earlier than usual.

Chapter 6

Self-Healing with Reiki

Using Reiki for self-healing involves taking responsibility for your own health and well-being. The word responsibility really means "being able to respond." In this case it means responding to your body's messages, learning from them and moving forward with a better understanding of what your body needs—and what you, as a whole, need in your life. It also means treating your body and your whole self with love and respect. Giving yourself a Reiki self-treatment can be a very important part of being loving to yourself, and I will describe how to do this later in this chapter.

Essentially, all healing is self-healing because whatever interventions take place, whether conventional medical methods or complementary therapies, it is the body's own repair and replication capabilities that carry out the healing. Reiki can be tremendously valuable in helping you to achieve optimum health, but it is not a cure-all. It will help to alleviate symptoms and relieve pain and discomfort, but it still needs a change of consciousness, a willingness on the part of the person receiving the Reiki to allow changes in lifestyle, in attitude and in ways of being, so that the healing can be completed and fully integrated into that person's life.

Even if you use Reiki on yourself every day but continue with any harmful habits or behaviors that are taking a toll on your physical, mental or emotional well-being, whatever you are doing that is causing you harm will continue to harm you. Initially you may well see a considerable improvement in your health, because

Reiki is wonderful, and it can potentially do the most miraculous and amazing things. But Reiki is not an impenetrable shield and it does not make you invincible! It involves you in your own healing, encouraging you to take responsibility for your own wholeness and health.

Being able to use Reiki on yourself for self-healing is one of the major advantages—and the main emphasis—of Reiki First Degree. As you start bringing Reiki into yourself regularly it begins the process of dislodging blockages and obstacles within your energetic system, slowly and systematically affecting deeper and deeper layers of blocked and stagnant energy caused by suppressed or buried negative and damaging thoughts, emotions, attitudes and beliefs.

When these blocks are dislodged and removed they come to the surface for attention. This often means that memories of past events suddenly come into your mind, or you start to have very vivid dreams. Occasionally you may even find that previous situations recur, so you might begin to feel that all those old problems you thought you had sorted out long ago have come back to plague you. But if they do, it is only to make you face up to them, and when you do they will soon disappear.

This is a necessary part of the process of letting go, and the memories, dreams or situations have surfaced to give you an opportunity to heal them and learn from them. Naturally this is an on-going process, as you cannot rid yourself of years of blocked or stagnant energy overnight. But as the process continues, over weeks, months and even years, you will gradually find that you feel better than you have ever felt before—lighter, more vital and energetic, less concerned about other people's opinions, more in touch with your own feelings and happier with yourself and your life.

INTENTION AND INVOCATION

Reiki does not need any complicated rituals before it will start to flow. All it takes is your intention to use it, which can be accompanied by a simple invocation such as "Let Reiki flow now for the highest and greatest good." Thoughts are an energy form and can be very powerful, especially with the force of intention behind them.

Actually, Reiki will begin to flow from the moment you first think of using it, so as you place your hands on whatever needs healing, it is already flowing. However, where and how Reiki flows is not up to you—you are merely a channel for this healing energy—because it is Divinely guided, so it goes where it is needed, not necessarily where the person using it, or the person receiving it, wants it. Having the intention that it should flow for the highest and greatest good therefore helps to get rid of the ego that might otherwise be involved.

For example, you might truly wish, with the best of intentions, to heal a friend's illness, but if it is for your friend's highest and greatest good for the physical symptoms to remain while they face up to the causative issues, then the Reiki will go to the causative levels—mental, emotional or spiritual. It may also bring some temporary relief of symptoms, but you can never guarantee what Reiki will do, because it is never under your control.

You therefore need to rid yourself of expectations as to outcome—which can be very hard, I know, because most of us in the Reiki community have a deep desire to help people. But please realize that by channeling Reiki you *are* helping people, even if that help does not turn out exactly the way you hoped it would.

MAKING A FRESH START

A Reiki initiation is a fresh start in life, and your first priority really needs to be self-healing, before you begin to use Reiki on other people, because when your own energies have been cleared you will be in a better position to help others. Remember the adage "physician, heal thyself?" Well, this is the major focus of Reiki at the First Degree level, and that means putting yourself first. It is about giving yourself the time to focus on your life, your thoughts, your emotions and your body; giving yourself time to listen to your body's messages and that inner voice that tells you when something feels "right."

Of course, in today's busy lives, finding time for yourself can be a challenge, but unless you are living exactly the way you want to live, as healthily as possible, you need to be willing to make some changes in your life—and giving yourself some time and space for the things you need could be the first of these changes.

It makes sense to take a good look at your life to see if it is helping or hindering you in achieving optimum holistic health. Are you eating a really healthy diet, or snatching fast food on the run to your next meeting? Are your major relationships—with partners, children, siblings, parents and close friends—healthy and loving or stressful and tense? Are you happy with whatever work you do, whether that's in external employment or in the home, or do you really long to do something else? Do you have time to indulge in hobbies and interests that add to your life, or are you always working or rushing around making everyone else's lives easier? Have you achieved some of your dreams and goals and expect to achieve even more, or have you given up the unequal struggle and settled for whatever you can get? Do you think life is wonderful, fun and a joy, or do you find it all too much of an effort and you cannot think why you bother?

Basically, the only person who has the power to change your life is *you*. Magazines and newspapers these days are full of articles on how to understand your motivations, make changes and improve your life, and there are several books recommended in the Further Reading section too, which should give you lots of ideas.

It also helps to clear out your life on a very practical level, so I would recommend a really good spring clean regardless of the season. Go through all your cupboards and drawers, shelves and wardrobes, old suitcases and boxes, attics and basements. At home—or even in your workplace, if possible—throw away, give away or sell *everything* that you don't love or don't use.

It may all sound like a lot of hard work, but you will get a real sense of achievement when you have done some clutter clearing—and you will find energy benefits, too. Things that should really have been discarded long ago, such as clothes you never wear, magazines you never read or kitchen gadgets that you have never used, all hold "old energy"—energy that reflects the time they were new. You may have moved on, but if you hold on to too many useless possessions they can hold you back energetically. If you throw out the old it rids your environment of stagnant, blocked energy, and leaves room for new energy to enter your life so that you really can make a fresh start.

THE IMPORTANCE OF DAILY SELF-TREATMENT

Being able to give yourself Reiki each day is a vital part of your own self-healing. Because Reiki works holistically, your use of it helps the whole of you—body, mind, emotions and spirit—to reach a state of harmony and balance. An essential part of this self-healing is giving yourself a daily self-treatment.

During your Reiki 1 course you should be shown the hand positions (usually about 12) for giving yourself a Reiki treatment, and your Reiki Master may also include some additional hand positions for certain conditions. I recommend that when self-treating, each hand position is held for between three and five minutes, so a full treatment would take somewhere between thirty-six minutes and an hour. This can obviously depend upon what time you have available, and if absolutely necessary the time for each hand position can be shortened to one or two minutes. A little Reiki is better than no Reiki at all and you can perhaps give yourself an extra-long treatment another day.

In terms of timing, there are CDs and tapes available of gentle music in three- or five-minute slots especially made for use when doing Reiki treatments, so those might be helpful. I find it easiest to count the seconds silently—it turns the treatment into a type of meditation and in any case I prefer to keep my eyes closed so I cannot see the clock, although I find its rhythmic ticking helps me to count the seconds at the right speed.

The more practice you get in self-treatment, the easier it will be to just let the energy dictate the time you need in each hand position, and even exactly where your hands should be placed. However, if you are always rushing your self-treatment, allowing yourself less and less time, perhaps you should ask yourself why. Why can you not spare about half an hour for yourself? Don't you feel you deserve it? Or are you living life at too hectic a pace? Are you giving your needs too little priority, rushing around after everyone else instead? Giving Reiki to yourself is a loving act and giving yourself some loving attention is not selfish. It is sensible. If you feel loved and cherished—even if it is only by yourself—then you will have more love to give to others, too.

Self-treatments can be carried out almost anywhere and at any time of day, but they are more comfortable if you are lying in bed or sitting in a comfortable chair so that your body and arms are well supported. For me, the best time is just after I have woken up in the morning—though I do set my alarm clock to ring again about 40 minutes later in case I get so relaxed that I drift back to sleep.

It is also really pleasant to do a self-treatment the last thing at night before you go to sleep, although if you are tired you probably will not get much past the fourth or fifth hand position before drifting off into peaceful slumber. Doing a Reiki self-treatment is therefore excellent if you have trouble getting to sleep or if you wake up in the middle of the night and cannot get back to sleep again.

Of course, your self-treatment does not always have to be at the same time each day—you can choose a point that is convenient to you, because it should be something you enjoy doing for yourself, not something you feel forced to do. You could try it just after the children have left for school or on your lunch break; it is even possible while sitting on a bus or train if you commute.

The benefits of giving yourself daily self-treatments are cumulative—the more Reiki you receive, the better Reiki is able to remove blockages and promote deep healing on all levels. Once it becomes a habit, you will probably find that you really miss it if for some reason you don't give yourself a treatment, because apart from its health benefits it is also a very pleasant, meditative experience.

One thing I need to point out is that when you are treating yourself you rarely get as much sensation in your hands as when you are treating other people. I have been self-treating since 1991, and unless I am treating particular areas of my body that are sore, aching or injured, I don't feel anything in my hands at all—and many of my students report the same thing. Don't worry—this does not mean the Reiki is not flowing; you will probably get other indications, anyway, such as feeling very relaxed.

If your hands do become hot, cold or tingly when treating specific areas, however, or if the part of your body that you are treating is experiencing similar sensations, this would indicate that more Reiki is required, so do please leave your hands in place until the sensation diminishes. There is no need to time the hand positions to the exact second. The timings are a rough guide, and there is no reason why you cannot have your hands in the same position for half an hour or more if you feel you need to.

HAND POSITIONS FOR A FULL SELF-TREATMENT

The Reiki hand positions for a self-treatment follow the chakras down the body, first down the front and then down the back, so it is quite easy to remember them, and once you have practiced them for a while it will become second nature. Most Reiki Masters teach 12 hand positions for both self-treatment and treatment of others—four on the head, four on the front of the body and four on the back of the body.

Each hand position should feel comfortable; otherwise you will not get the full benefit in terms of relaxation. Your hands should be laid gently on your body in the order shown on pages 86–92, and it is usual to keep your fingers close together, with the thumbs also close to the hand. This seems to help focus the energy more efficiently than if the fingers and thumbs are wide apart, perhaps because the hand chakra is deep in the center of the palm, although Reiki does come out of your fingertips and the backs of your hands too.

You will notice that each hand is placed on a different side of the body. Treating each side of the body equally helps balance the energies, encouraging a good flow of *Ki* around the body's energy system. However, if you have any disability or injury that prevents you from using two hands, such as a broken arm, a stroke or an amputation, then you can place one hand on one side and *intend*, or visualize, that the other hand is in a complementary pos-ition on the other side. Energy follows intentional thought, so the Reiki will flow through appropriate parts of your energy body—even if an arm or leg is amputated, its subtle energy counterparts are still there—and will then flow into wherever you intend it to go.

You will also notice that the treatment is started at the head. The first three hand positions then focus the Reiki toward the crown and third-eye chakras. The treatment then works down the front of the body, over the throat, heart, solar plexus, sacral and root chakras. Energy can flow into and out of the body through any of the chakras, but when it flows into the crown chakra first and from there down through the rest of the energy body, it seems to enable the Reiki to move more easily into the other chakras, as well as having a gentler, more calming and relaxing effect. If the energy is taken in first through the root chakra or the feet, while it is in no way harmful to do Reiki that way, it tends to have a more vibrant and energizing effect, which some people find slightly agitating, so I don't generally recommend this.

PREPARING FOR SELF-TREATMENT

Before you start your self-treatment, it is a good idea to spend a few moments just gently centering yourself by breathing deeply and evenly, and allowing your body to relax. Generally I recommend that you close your eyes, and as you raise your hands to place them in the first position over the eyes, think and *intend* that you are beginning a self-treatment, and think and *intend* that the Reiki flows into you for your highest and greatest good.

Hand Positions for the Front of the Body

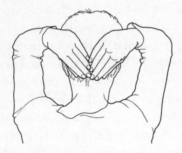 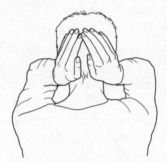

1a. The back of the head Both hands next to each other at the back of the head pointing downward with the fingertips at the base of the skull.

1b. As an alternative you can place your hands next to each other at the back of the head, with the heel of each hand level with the base of the skull, fingertips pointing toward the crown.

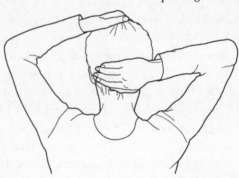

1c. Another alternative, which is particularly comforting, but is not normally a part of the traditional hand positions, is one hand on the crown of the head and the other covering the back of the head.

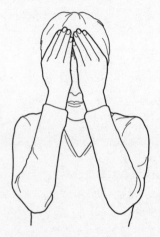

2. The eyes *One hand held loosely over each eye with the heel of each hand placed on your cheekbones, fingertips on your brow.*

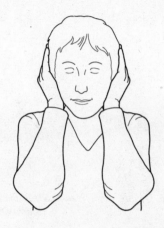

3. The ears *One hand held loosely cupped over each ear with the heel of each hand placed a fraction below the earlobe and fingertips pointing upward toward the top of the head.*

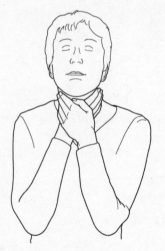

4a. The throat *One hand on top of the other covering the throat.*

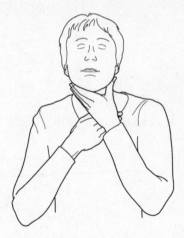

4b. Or *one hand at the top of the chest and the other covering the throat.*

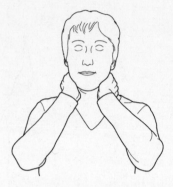

4c. Or *one hand on each side of the neck—it is okay to have the heels of the hands touching or slightly apart.*

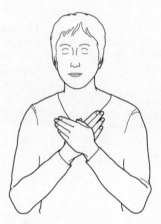

5a. The chest *Both hands crossed in the center of the chest over the heart chakra.*

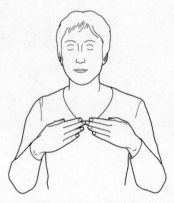

5b. Or *one hand on each side of the chest, very slightly above each breast. The fingertips can touch in the center or be slightly apart.*

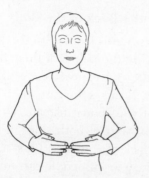

6. The solar plexus *One hand on each side of the body covering the solar plexus (midriff). Again, the fingertips can touch in the center or be slightly apart.*

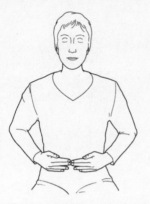

7. The waist *One hand on each side of the body, fingers pointing toward each other at about the same level as your navel, which can be either very slightly above or below your natural waistline.*

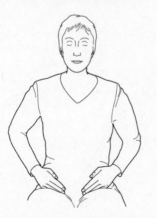

8. The pelvic area *One hand on each side of the body, fingers pointing downward but slightly diagonally in a V-shape sloping toward the pelvic area.*

Hand Positions for the Back of the Body

When positioning the hands for the back of the body, some people find difficulty in having the palms of their hands flat against their body, particularly if they have any stiffness in their wrists or fingers, such as with arthritis. If this is the case, then you can place the *back* of your hand against your body instead. The palm chakra, like all other chakras, spreads out of both sides of the hand so the Reiki will flow out of the back of your hand just as well, if that is what it needs to do. For quite a lot of people this makes hand positions 10 and 11 much more comfortable.

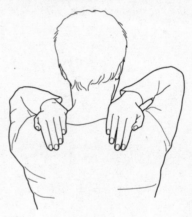

9a. The shoulders Place one hand on top of each shoulder, or if this is uncomfortable, try 9b.

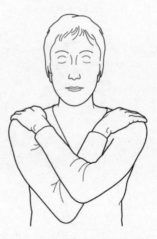

9b. Alternatively, place one hand on top of each shoulder by crossing your arms in front of your chest.

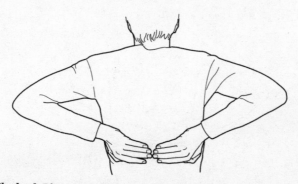

10a. The back *Place one hand on each side of the back, palms flat on the back, preferably midway between the shoulders and the waist, but if this is difficult then as high above your waist as you can comfortably manage.*

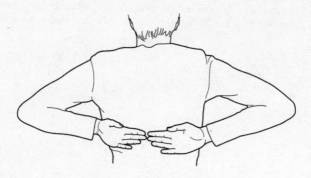

10b. If it is uncomfortable *to place your palms flat on your back, put the back of each hand against your back instead, as high above your waist as you can comfortably manage.*

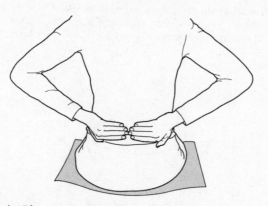

11a. The waist *Place one hand on each side of your body, with palms flat against your back, with your fingers pointing toward each other and your thumbs tucked into your natural waistline.*

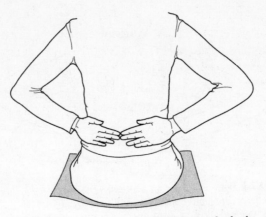

11b. If it is uncomfortable *to place your palms flat on your back, then place the back of each hand against your back instead, with the fingertips pointing toward each other, this time with your little fingers tucked into your natural waistline.*

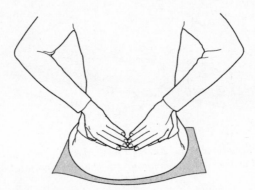

11c. As an alternative, *you can place your hands with the heel of each hand at waist level and the fingertips pointing slightly downward in a V shape. (You can also do this as an extra hand position, if you have lower back pain).*

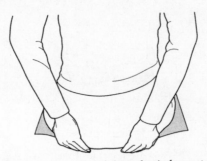

12. The buttocks *Place one hand on each buttock—it does not matter which way the hands are facing as long as you're comfortable.*

Additional Hand Positions

It is *optional* to give Reiki to the thighs, knees, calves, ankles and feet, or to the upper arms, elbows, forearms, wrists, hands or fingers. Naturally, if you have a health problem in any of those places it makes sense to treat it. For any of the optional hand positions on the legs and feet you can have one hand on each leg— for example, left hand on left knee, right hand on right knee. Alternatively, you can place one hand under and one hand on top of each position moving down the whole of one leg and foot and then down the other leg and foot, moving from thigh to knee to calf to ankle to foot (see sample illustration below).

Example, the knees:

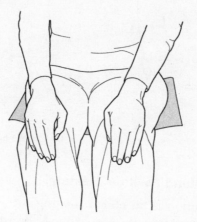

a. You can either place one hand on each knee.

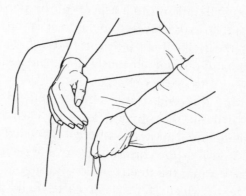

b. Or you can place one hand underneath and one hand on top of one knee at a time.

If you wish to treat your arms and hands, it is probably easiest and most comfortable to do them one at a time, although it is just about possible to treat both arms together. Work downward from the upper arm to the elbow, the forearm, the wrist and the hand.

Example, the elbows:

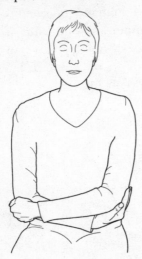

a. You can either place one hand on each elbow.   *b. Or you can place one hand on each elbow, one at a time.*

What Is Each Hand Position Treating?

Every hand position is, in effect, treating the whole of the body, because the Reiki flows into and around the whole subtle energy and physical bodies through the meridians. It is also affecting the mental, emotional and spiritual aspects of the person, healing or "wholing," and bringing everything into harmony and balance. However, as the Reiki flows into the body of the person being treated, each hand position obviously allows the Reiki to move into particular areas with greater effect.

The following three illustrations give a general guide to what *might* be treated on the physical level by each hand position. However, the Reiki will always go where it is needed, and this is not under your control or the conscious control of the person you are treating. Also, because the Reiki can flow through the meridians of the energy body, which connect all parts, Reiki applied at the shoulder could equally well end up in the feet.

Hand positions 1, 2 and 3 work together to cover the brain, nervous system, pineal and pituitary glands, endocrine system, head, face and eyes.

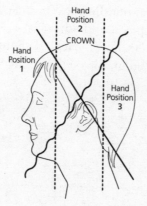

Hand positions 1–3.

Hand position 4 covers ears, nose, mouth, teeth, neck, throat, thyroid and parathyroid.

Hand position 5 covers heart and circulatory system, lungs and respiratory system, thymus gland and immune system, arms and hands.

Hand position 6 covers liver, spleen, gallbladder, stomach, small intestine, digestive system, pancreas and muscles.

Hand position 7 covers kidneys, lower digestive organs, urinary tract, prostate, lower back and reproductive system.

Hand position 8 covers skeleton, skin, blood, large intestine, elimination system, adrenal gland, pelvis, hips, legs and feet.

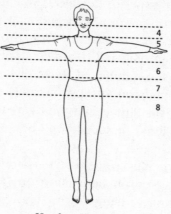

Hand positions 4–8.

Hand position 9 covers shoulders, arms and hands.

Hand position 10 covers upper back, thymus gland, heart and lungs.

Hand position 11 covers middle back, muscles, pancreas, digestive system, liver, kidneys, spleen and adrenals.

Hand position 12 covers lower back, skeleton, skin, elimination system, reproductive system, hips, legs and feet.

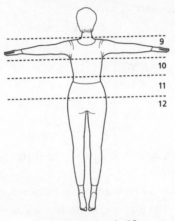

Hand positions 9–12.

OTHER WAYS OF USING REIKI ON YOURSELF

Although doing a self-treatment every day is an excellent practice to promote self-healing, don't feel that it is the only way to give yourself Reiki. Reiki can be as flexible as you are, so you can place your hands anywhere on your body and allow the energy to flow through you almost anywhere, at any time, throughout the day.

You can add to your daily self-treatment as often as you like, giving yourself five or ten minutes of Reiki, or longer if you like, by just placing your hands on an appropriately convenient place—your chest, solar plexus, stomach or thighs are usually the easiest—and intending that Reiki should flow always for your highest and greatest good.

The point is, if you have some time to spare give yourself Reiki. It does not require any conscious effort on your part. You don't even *have* to be sitting or lying down. Simply put your hands on any part of your body that you can comfortably reach and allow the

Reiki to flow. You can then feel that you are doing yourself some good even when you are just being a couch potato!

GIVING YOURSELF "FIRST AID" TREATMENT

There is no need to give yourself a full self-treatment every time you have a headache or cut your finger. Although a full self-treatment is always beneficial it is not always essential, so if you have a stiff neck or aching shoulders, treat them. If you have a headache or sore eyes, treat them. If you fall and graze your knee or trap your fingers in a door, treat them. All you need to do is *intend* that the Reiki should flow and it will. If your injury is more serious, it makes sense to seek medical help or advice—but you can give yourself Reiki while you wait for professional attention (but see the cautions below).

As well as giving yourself Reiki for first aid remember to give yourself lots of Reiki if you are ill. You cannot "overdose" on Reiki, so if you are feeling ill just place your hands on yourself anywhere that is comfortable and let the Reiki keep flowing for as many hours as you like. It will accelerate your body's own healing processes and help it to fight off whatever "bug" you have caught. Initially it may exacerbate your symptoms—because many of the distressing symptoms we experience are actually the effects of the body's activities to fight off infection—but it will shorten the length of time you feel ill, which has to be a good thing.

TIMES FOR CAUTION

There are very few times when it might be sensible to exercise caution when giving Reiki but there are a couple of issues to look out for. If you have the misfortune to chop off a toe or finger in an accident, for example, then the obvious thing is to pack the missing part carefully and get to a hospital as quickly as possible so that it can be reattached surgically.

The caution here is that Reiki accelerates healing, so if you apply Reiki directly to the hand or foot in this case, the natural healing process of closing the wound will quickly begin to take place. There has been at least one case I know of where the severed finger could not be reattached, even though the man in question went straight to the hospital after the accident. The hospital could not understand why he had not gone there sooner as the wound had healed so much it looked as though it had happened several days before.

In a case like this, by all means give yourself Reiki but not directly on the injured part. Instead, place a hand on your heart chakra or over your kidneys to help with the pain and shock, and although the Reiki will flow throughout the body, including to the injury, it will do so in a much gentler way, so the healing effect will not be so dramatic.

The same caution applies in the case of a bad break of an arm, leg, wrist or ankle, etc. This will probably need professional setting, and again, if the healing process has already begun this could cause problems because the bone(s) might not be aligned properly. Reiki your heart chakra or adrenal glands to deal with the pain and shock rather than placing your hand directly on the break, until after the bone has been set and put in a cast. After that, give it as much as possible, and it will mend much more quickly.

I have actually known a number of people—all Reiki Masters— who have broken bones and managed to heal them completely within hours, using Reiki. So in the case of a straightforward break this is definitely possible—but it does take a great deal of belief in Reiki to trust its process, so I would always advise people to get professional medical help.

QUICK ENERGY BOOSTS

Sometimes when your energy is running low because you have been busy or had a stressful day, you could do with a bit of a boost, so I came up with this technique, which seems to work well:

The Ten-minute Top-up

1. First, *intend* that the Reiki should flow for your highest and greatest good (that is, just thinking that you want to use Reiki will activate it). Place one hand over your eyes, with the palm facing and touching your face and the other hand at the back of your head, palm against the head. (It does not matter which hand is where—for example left at front or back.) Hold your

hands in this position for two and a half minutes—counting to 150 is the way I keep a check on the time, but of course you can continue for a longer period if you want to.

2. Next, place one hand on your throat and the other hand on the center of your chest, again for about two and a half minutes.

3. Then place one hand on your solar plexus and the other one on your navel for another two and a half minutes.

4. Finally, place one hand on the top of your head, over your crown chakra, and the other one on your root chakra, either on your bottom (or underneath it if you are sitting down), or with your hand between your legs for two and a half minutes.

The Wake-up

Another useful tip is a hand position that works on hangovers. It is also good as a quick "wake-up" when you are feeling tired but need to do some tasks. To do this, place both hands, one hand crossed over the other, on the crown of your head. *Intend* that the Reiki should flow and keep your hands in that position for at least five minutes.

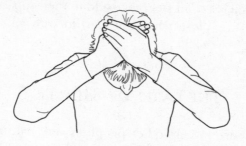

Hand position for wake-up.

These are the basics of self-healing with Reiki, although you will find other ideas in later chapters, and do feel free to experiment. The classic self-treatment is a good structure to start with, but of course you can add to it. For example, at the end of the 12 hand positions I always treat each foot for a few minutes. I hold it between both hands and then finish with some gentle massage, which I find helps to "ground" my energy and helps me to become alert again after enjoying the deeply relaxed state during the treatment.

Chapter 7

Treating Family and Friends

Although the major emphasis of Reiki First Degree is self-healing, most people want to try out their Reiki on other people too. It would be inadvisable to set up as a professional Reiki Practitioner right from the word go because obviously you will need plenty of practice in order to develop your knowledge and confidence. I always recommend that anyone wishing to practice professionally should take Reiki Second Degree to add to their capabilities, but to begin with let's explore what you can do with your Reiki First Degree skills.

THE LABEL OF "HEALER"

Having the desire to help other people is very natural and being able to treat people with Reiki is a very pleasurable experience. However, there can be a problem, and that is the label of "healer" which some people will attach to you. The word implies a certain status and ability and it is very easy to get caught up in the illusion of it all and to enjoy the sense of esteem it can give you. But even if people do call us "healers" it is not a factual description.

The body does all its own healing, and because we are channels for Reiki that means we are able to act as catalysts, helping to get the healing process kick-started by delivering, through our hands, some healing energy. Actually, the more we push our own ego out of the way, the more we are able to go with the energy and let it direct us and the stronger the flow of energy becomes. But it is important to remember that *we* don't do any healing. Reiki does—or at least, it is the Reiki that helps the person to heal themself.

WHAT IS A REIKI TREATMENT?

For many people, their first contact with Reiki is through receiving a Reiki treatment from a friend, a member of their family or a professional Reiki Practitioner. Normally a Reiki treatment takes about an hour and is carried out with the client remaining fully clothed (except for shoes) and tucked up comfortably with a blanket and pillows, usually on a therapy couch. (I am using the words "client" and "Practitioner" for simplification, but I mean anyone receiving and giving Reiki. Other terms like "patient" and "healer" are more emotive, and therefore I prefer not to use them.)

The treatment starts with the client lying on his or her back and the Practitioner's hands are placed gently on the body in specific places and will normally be kept still for a few minutes—there is no pressure, massage or manipulation unless the Reiki is being combined with another therapy. The responses during the treatment vary considerably. Some clients experience feelings of heat or tingling as the Reiki flows through them, or certain parts of their body might feel cold, especially after the Practitioner's hands have moved away. Usually the client feels very relaxed and peaceful as the energy flows through their body, and many clients drift off to sleep and have to be gently roused when it is time to turn over to lie on their front for the rest of the treatment.

However, clients can sometimes become quite emotional as the Reiki begins to break down old patterns and blockages and bring them to the surface. They may laugh out loud or even shed some tears, or their legs or arms may suddenly jerk even while they are asleep. It is important to tell the client before the treatment that these reactions are possible and to reassure them that they are perfectly normal—they are just blocked or stagnant energy being released in different ways from the body.

Sometimes after the treatment has ended clients may experience a shift in consciousness, a realization of the underlying causes of any problems they have been having, whether those problems have to do with their physical health, their relationships, or their job, etc.

This is an important part of healing, and if the client wants to talk about it with you, that is fine, but this is where the boundaries can become blurred between being a friend or family member and being a healer or counselor. Whatever issues are raised it is important to remain nonjudgmental, and to be as comforting and supportive as possible.

If talking with clients in this way is something you don't feel very comfortable with, you might find it useful to take a short counseling course or read some books about the counseling process. If you believe the person needs much more support, you could gently and tactfully suggest that they talk things over with a friend, a counselor or a family therapist, for example.

Please remember, though, that if you are treating someone, even if it is a close friend or a member of your family, they may regard you differently—as a health professional—so your client is entitled to expect your complete confidentiality. It is essential *never* to talk to other people about any clients or their treatments, unless you need advice on how to handle a particular situation. In that case you could contact your Reiki Master and discuss the case, while preserving your client's anonymity by not revealing their name, or any personal details that might identify them.

Occasionally in the days immediately following a treatment some people experience something called a "healing crisis," which is usually just a short period when they have temporary physical symptoms such as a sudden cold as the Reiki energy works through the blockages and the body does its best to get rid of them. I always tell clients about this possibility and encourage them to drink plenty of water during the next few days after a treatment, as this helps to flush any toxins out of the body in a natural way.

Receiving a Reiki treatment is great for anybody whatever their age. Babies and small children usually love Reiki, although they don't often want to stay still long enough for a full treatment, and since they are so much smaller than an adult they don't need as much Reiki anyway. It is far easier to treat them casually, just allowing the Reiki to flow while you hold them or when they sit on your knee.

Pregnant women usually find Reiki very soothing for themselves and their unborn child, and it can be really beneficial to both mother and baby to give Reiki during the birth process. Otherwise, adults of any age will find a Reiki treatment very helpful with any health or stress-related problems and, of course, people don't have to be ill to benefit from a Reiki treatment. It is lovely just to relax and be nurtured for a while.

EQUIPMENT

You don't really need any expensive equipment in order to give Reiki to someone—all you need is your hands. However, if you intend to carry out any Reiki treatments, it is sensible to have something suitable for people to lie on. The best option, if you can afford it, is a therapy couch, and there are several different types on the market. Costs vary depending upon which country you live in, but in the U.K. prices start at around £150 to £350 for portable couches, some of which have adjustable leg heights. Similar ones are available in the U.S. for around $350 to $600. However, hydraulically operated static couches can go up to several thousand pounds (or dollars). You may find one secondhand, which will be cheaper, but the best source of information about suitable therapy couches is the Yellow Pages, or advertisements in a health magazine.

One thing to watch for is that many therapy couches are made for the massage market, so they are low enough to allow the therapist to bend over a client and exert some pressure. When doing Reiki you need a couch that allows you to stand beside your client with your hands held at a comfortable height, which is usually somewhere around the middle of your chest, but no lower than your waist. Of course, your hands will be supported on your client's body, but nevertheless it can be uncomfortable to hold your hands still for about five minutes if you have to bend your back to reach. However, you will not need to invest in an expensive couch unless you intend to become a Practitioner, so in the meantime there are other inexpensive alternatives.

First of all, you could use your dining table. These are usually about the right height. If it is sturdy and long enough, you could place some thick foam on top and cover it with a sheet. Another alternative could be a heavy-duty decorating table with foam on top. The heavy-duty models are made of stronger materials, and have wooden braces that can be screwed into place to make the whole thing solid.

If you are reasonably agile, you could do treatments with a person lying on a cot or chaise longue with you sitting on the floor with your legs under the bed. It is also possible to do treatments with people lying on the floor or on a conventional divan bed, but while these might be reasonably relaxing for the person you are treating, they can be very uncomfortable for you unless you are used to sitting cross-legged on the floor. It is also possible to give someone a Reiki treatment while they are sitting in a chair, and I discuss that later in this chapter.

In each of the above cases, you will also need several pillows, pillowcases, fitted sheets (stretch toweling is best) to fit over the therapy couch or over the foam layer if you are using that, and a soft blanket to cover the client.

PREPARATION

If you are going to give someone a full Reiki treatment, I would recommend that you wait until you have completed your own 21-day clearing and cleansing process, and have done plenty of self-treatments. Once you are ready to begin, remember that it is important that anyone you treat should come into a comfortable, safe and supportive environment, and they also need you to behave in a professional manner, even if they know you really well. Before you give anyone a Reiki treatment it is important that you should prepare yourself and the space in which the treatment is to take place.

Personal Preparation

There are two priorities for your self-preparation—energetic protection and cleansing. When I was originally taught Reiki in 1991, no mention was made of either, other than ensuring that we washed our hands before starting a treatment. However, over the years I have come to realize that some further preparation *is* necessary, and certainly since 2000, when I learned Dr. Usui's original techniques, I have recognized that there was considerable emphasis on self-cleansing in the Japanese tradition.

Self-cleansing

The first priority for your own sake, and especially for the comfort of your client, is to pay particular attention to personal hygiene. So in addition to washing your hands (and probably brushing your teeth) before treating anybody, you need to ensure that you—and your clothes—are clean and fresh. There is nothing worse than having someone leaning over you with garlic breath or smelling of sweat or stale tobacco. You should also remove your watch and any metal jewelry (except for a wedding ring), or anything else that might catch on a client's clothing, or jangle distractingly.

Energetic Protection

It is just as important to be energetically cleansed, and there are various methods detailed in chapter 15, which I would recommend that you try, such as the *Hatsurei-ho* technique. As you become more sensitive and intuitive, which often happens after taking a Reiki attunement, it can be a good idea to start protecting yourself energetically and psychically.

Psychic protection is dealt with more fully in chapter 14, but the simplest method is to create an energetic barrier by imagining your aura filled with Reiki, and if you wish, you can see its outer edge like a translucent eggshell made of energy. Imagine the Reiki flowing out of your hands, filling the eggshell with healing white light, and *intend* that the Reiki protect you from any negativity or harm, so any negative or harmful energies within your aura will be cleansed and released by the Reiki, and the outer edge of your aura will only permit love, light and Reiki to enter.

During a treatment your client will be inside your auric field, so doing this will mean that both you and your client will be surrounded by protective Reiki, and any negative energies released by the client during the treatment will not stick to your energy field, but will be healed and transformed by the Reiki. Of course you can set up a protective energy field around yourself any time, not just when doing a Reiki treatment: before going shopping in a city center or if you are visiting a hospital, or anywhere else that could hold negative energies.

Preparing the Space

Whatever kind of space you use should be clean and tidy, and you can further prepare it by cleansing it with Reiki. Just sit quietly for a few moments, resting your hands on your thighs, palms facing upward, and then allow Reiki to flow through your hands and out into the room, *intending* that the Reiki should cleanse it of any negative energies. Visualize the Reiki flowing like a soft white mist all over the room, especially into all the corners.

Set up the therapy couch if you have one, and place clean pillows and a soft blanket ready, perhaps burning some incense or essential oils to fill the room with a pleasant smell. (Some people are sensitive to certain smells, so don't do this until you have checked with the client.) If you plan to play some relaxing music get the CD or tape ready in the machine and test it for volume before you start. Also ensure that the room is at an appropriate temperature and that there will be no interruptions from telephones, children, pets or other distractions.

Preparing Your Client

Lots of people are a bit nervous before having their first Reiki treatment (and you might be equally nervous at first), so always spend a little time beforehand talking to them about what Reiki is, and what to expect during the treatment, including where you will be placing your hands. Explain to them that you will not be touching any "personal" areas, such as genitals or women's breasts. They usually find it reassuring when they realize they can remain fully clothed, except for taking off their shoes, as people are often self-conscious about revealing their bodies.

Also tell them what sorts of experience they may have, such as feeling sensations of warmth, heat or tingling where your hands are placed, or sensing energy flowing around their body. Explain that they will probably become very relaxed but might feel a bit emotional, so reassure them that if they need to laugh or cry this is quite normal and it is also absolutely okay with you, and they don't need to feel embarrassed.

Talk to them about the reason they have come for a treatment, and give them a chance to ask questions. Point out to them that they don't need to do anything consciously in order for the Reiki to flow into them, other than being willing to let it happen.

People receiving Reiki should take off their shoes, watch, glasses and any metal jewelry (there is no need to ask anyone to remove a wedding ring), but should otherwise remain fully clothed. When clients are lying on their back at the beginning of the treatment, a pillow should be placed under their head and another one under their knees. When they turn over to lie on their front, move the pillow from under their knees and place it under the ankles, to take the pressure off their back.

Sometimes putting a soft blanket over the client helps to make them feel nurtured and more relaxed, and it also prevents them from feeling cold, as their body cools down when they are lying still or when negative energy is being released during the treatment.

It is important that both you and your client should enjoy the treatment, so before you start make sure that both of you are comfortable, that the therapy couch is at a comfortable height for you, and that the client is warm enough.

I usually explain to clients that it is preferable for them to close their eyes, so they can fully relax, and I discourage talking or asking questions during the treatment; although if a client is initially nervous I will, of course, continue to answer in as gentle and supportive a manner as I can. However, I find that by the time I have reached the third hand position (or even earlier) their speech becomes slurred as they enter a state of deep relaxation, after which they generally go quiet, often drifting off to sleep. I find that playing soft, relaxing music—classical or "New Age"—often helps people to feel at ease, although you should check this with your client.

HAND POSITIONS FOR THE TREATMENT OF OTHERS

When doing a treatment, your hands are always used with the fingers closed, and the thumb close to the hand. The most usual form of full Reiki treatment in the West is based on 12 hand positions on the head and body.

Each position is normally held for about five minutes with the option of leaving the hands on longer in any position where you can feel that there is still a lot of Reiki flowing (for example heat, coldness, tingling, buzzing sensations, and so on), which would indicate that the area still needs more energy.

Some Reiki Masters teach a slightly different structure for the treatment, with up to six hand positions on the head and neck, and up to ten hand positions on the front of the body, including the legs and feet, and another ten on the back of the body, again including the legs and feet. This gives a total of 26 hand positions, with those on the head and body being held for about five minutes and those on the legs and feet being held for two or three minutes.

Even though I now know and have tried out the 68 hand positions that Dr. Usui used, in almost every case I continue to use the 12 hand positions I was originally taught. They allow Reiki to flow into every chakra, and around the whole physical and energy body, so even when I feel strongly drawn to give Reiki to some extra places, I just add them to the flow and rhythm of the traditional Western treatment.

It takes just over an hour if each position is held for five minutes, allowing a few minutes for the client to turn over so that their back can be treated. If more hand positions are used, it will take longer—about an hour and a half. It is therefore important that both you and your client should be comfortable. Holding the hands still for any length of time can be a strain if you don't have the Reiki couch, or other suitable equipment, at the right height.

It is usual to start with clients lying on their back with their arms at their sides, and the Practitioner standing or sitting behind their head for the first five hand positions. The hands are supposed to rest *gently* on the person's body, so be careful not to exert any pressure.

Most people find the gentle placing of the hands on the body very reassuring, but some people really cannot bear to be touched. You can therefore hold your hands above the body in the auric field at a height that is comfortable for you, and the Reiki will still flow into the client. This can also be useful for treating areas of the body where some form of injury means even the lightest pressure might be painful. However, holding your hands in the aura above the body without support can be tiring, so pay special attention to your stance or how you are seated to ensure that you are as comfortable as possible.

Some people, when they first start doing Reiki, are reluctant to place their hands on the client's body, feeling that it is in some way intrusive, so they barely allow their hands to touch the body, resulting in a hesitant, "fluttering" feeling that most clients don't like. If the hands are placed lightly but confidently, this helps to give the client a feeling of security, and as none of the hand positions is "intimate" there is no invasion of privacy.

Be very gentle when the hands are moved from one position to another, and move one hand at a time, if possible, so that you have continuity of contact. For hand positions 6 through 8, you will need to stand or sit at one side of the person being treated.

When you have finished treating the front of the body you will need to gently rouse the client (who is usually deeply relaxed at this stage) and ask them to turn over onto the front. Again, make sure they are comfortable, and help them to turn over if necessary, adjusting the pillows so that the head rests comfortably and the other pillow is placed under the ankles. Their arms don't have to be by their sides when they are lying on their front, so allow them to position them in any way they like. It is also a good idea to tell them that if they need to, they can alter their position. Sometimes people bravely stay in the same position despite being in considerable discomfort, because they think they are expected to.

When the client is settled again, the treatment can continue. Hand position 9, on the shoulders, is especially good for people who hold a lot of tension in their shoulders, which is probably most of us. You then progress down one side of the body for hand positions 10 through 12.

Treatment Alternatives

If the person is unable to lie on their stomach for the second part of the treatment, for example a pregnant woman, she can lie on her side instead. It is then more comfortable for you to sit at the side of the therapy couch facing her back, to carry out the rest of the treatment.

Should you ever need to treat anyone who cannot lie down at all, then the treatment can fairly easily be carried out with them sitting in a chair. If so, make sure that the client's legs are uncrossed, and that both feet are on the floor (or other support), as this enables the energy to flow most effectively. You can stand or sit behind them for the head positions, and then sit or kneel at their side for the hand positions on the front of the body.

If they are sitting on something like a dining chair, then the back-of-the-body hand positions are also relatively easy. However, if they can only sit in an armchair or a wheelchair, and are unable to lean forward a little, you can adapt the treatment to suit them. Either spend extra time on the front of the body or place your hands on the back of the chair in places that roughly correspond to the back-of-the-body hand positions; Reiki is a high vibrational energy, so it can easily go through the back of a chair.

Before You Start

When you have made sure your client is comfortable, it is time to make your own preparations. Spend a few minutes centering yourself by breathing deeply and evenly, and allowing your body to relax. I would then recommend that if you have not already done so, you carry out either the Dry Brushing or Reiki Shower self-cleansing techniques outlined in Chapter 15, after which you are ready to "tune in" to the Reiki by *intending* that it should flow.

You might like to invoke the Reiki silently by saying to yourself "I am now starting a full Reiki treatment on [name of person] and wish Reiki to flow into him/her for his/her highest and greatest good." This is not strictly necessary, as when you raise your hands to start the treatment, your thoughts have already been acted upon, and the Reiki will have started to flow, but it reaffirms your intentions.

Hand Positions for Treating the Front of the Body

The first five hand positions are carried out with the Practitioner either standing or sitting behind the client's head.

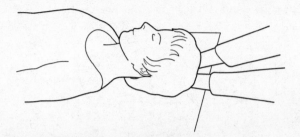

1. The back of the head *Very gently place both hands beneath the head, palms upward (sometimes it is easiest to do this one hand at a time, but take care not to pull their hair), so that your little fingers are touching each other and your fingertips are roughly level with the base of the skull. Remain in this position for 3 to 5 minutes, then gently and slowly slide both hands out at the same time, allowing the client's head to rest back on the pillow. Move your hands to position 2.*

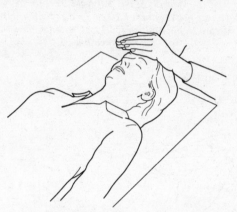

2. The eyes *Place one slightly cupped hand over each eye, with the heel of each hand resting gently on the brow, but make sure that the fingertips do not touch the face— keep them at least 5 cm (2 in) away. After 3 to 5 minutes, move the hands one at a time to position 3.*

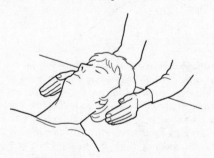

3. The ears *Place one slightly cupped hand over each ear, with the heel of each hand resting gently against the side of the head so that the fingertips are roughly level with each earlobe. Again, make sure the fingertips don't touch the face—leave them at least 5 cm (2 in) away. After 3 to 5 minutes, move the hands one at a time to position 4.*

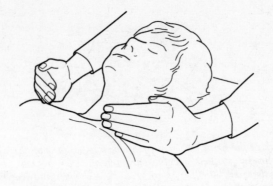

4. The neck Place one hand on each side of the neck, with palms facing the neck, and with your little fingers resting gently on top of the client's shoulders. Your fingers should not touch the person's neck, as this can make them feel very constricted, and even unsafe. Make sure there is at least 10 cm (4 in) between your hands and the client's neck. Remain in this position for 3 to 5 minutes, then move the hands one at a time to position 5.

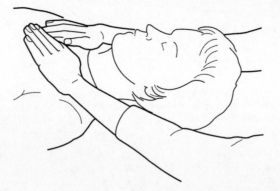

5. The chest Place your hands in a V shape at the top of the chest. The heel of each hand can rest gently on the person's collarbone, and the hand can be held flat on the chest this time, with fingertips pointing diagonally toward the breastbone in the center of the chest. If you are treating a female, be aware that it is neither appropriate nor necessary to have your hands directly on the breasts, so if you have long hands or the woman has particularly high breasts, you may need to pull your hands back a little. Hold your hands in this position for 3 to 5 minutes, then gently remove them, and move around to the side of the client.

The next three positions are carried out with the Practitioner standing or sitting on one side of the client. Ensure that you can comfortably hold each hand position for between 3 and 5 minutes, without having to stretch too much or press too hard on the client's body. Adjust your body appropriately, either by standing with your legs slightly apart with the knees soft, as in a t'ai chi or chi kung stance, or by sitting on a chair. (A chair on wheels, but without arms, is excellent, because this allows for minimal disturbance as you can wheel yourself along between hand positions, rather than having to reposition the chair.) If you are treating someone on the floor, sit cross-legged.

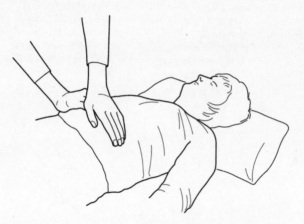

6. The solar plexus Place one hand in front of the other flat on the body (resting gently, but without putting pressure on the client), with fingertips pointing away from you, on the solar plexus (between the breasts and the waist), so that one hand is on the left side of the body and the other is on the right side. Hold this position for 3 to 5 minutes (it is okay to reposition your hands occasionally, swapping them over to different sides so that you don't get too tired), then move them one at a time to position 7.

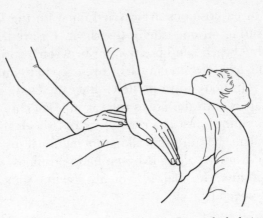

7. The waist *Place one hand in front of the other flat on the body (resting gently, but without putting pressure on the client), with fingertips pointing away from you, on the waist, so that one hand is on the left side of the body and the other is on the right side. Hold this position for 3 to 5 minutes (it is okay to reposition your hands occasionally, swapping them over to different sides so that you don't get too tired), then move them one at a time to position 8.*

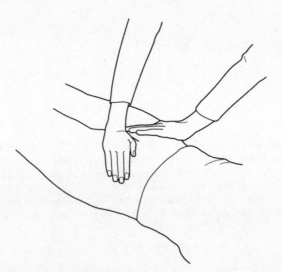

8a. The pelvic area—female *The hand positions for male and female vary slightly, in order to show sensitivity with regard to the genitals. For female clients, hold your hands in a V shape, with the point of the V being toward the pubic bone. This is most comfortably achieved as shown in the illustration. For example, if the client's head is on your right, then the heel of your right hand is level with her left hip bone and the fingertips are pointing diagonally toward the pubic bone. The fingertips of your left hand are pointing diagonally toward and level with her right hip. (Any other configuration of the hands tends to be uncomfortable to hold, and to be more intrusive to the client.) Hold this position for 3 to 5 minutes, then take your hands away.*

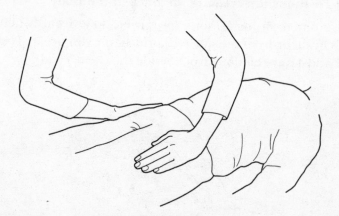

8b. The pelvic area—male In order to show sensitivity, and to avoid contact with the male genitalia, it is usual to place one hand on each hip bone, as shown in the illustration. Again, it is more comfortable for you to have one hand with the fingertips pointing to the right, and one hand with the fingertips pointing to the left. Hold this position for 3 to 5 minutes and then take your hands away. You may at this point start treating the front of the legs and feet, if needed.

Preparing to Work on the Back

When you have completed the first eight hand positions, which cover the head and the front of the body (plus the front of the legs and feet if necessary), you will need to ask your client to turn over onto their stomach. The person will probably be very relaxed at this stage, and may even be asleep, so it is important to be kind and supportive. Very gently pat or stroke their shoulder, speak their name softly, and ask them to turn over. Assist them if they need this, and ensure that you reposition the pillow that had been under their knees—move it so that it is now under their ankles.

Ensure that their head is comfortable—if you have a therapy couch with a face cradle (and the toweling-covered sponge ring that goes over this to make it more comfortable) then the client can use this, but sometimes people don't like to feel so constricted. The head can be held on one side, or it can rest on an arm—just let the client find a position that suits them, and when they are settled again, start the treatment of the back of the body.

Hand Positions for Treating the Back of the Body

Hand position 9a (or 9b and 9c) can be done from behind the client's head, or from the side (9d), whichever you prefer. Positions 10, 11 and 12 are all done from beside the client's body.

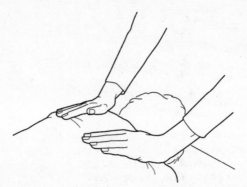

9a. The shoulders *Both shoulders can be treated at the same time, or separately (see 9b and 9c). If you choose to sit or stand behind the client's head, place one hand on each shoulder so that the heel of each hand rests on the shoulder, and the fingertips are pointing down the back. Hold this position for 3 to 5 minutes, then gently remove your hands and move around to the side of the client's body for hand position 10.*

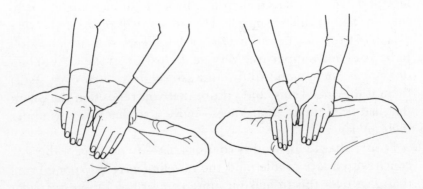

Or 9b and 9c. *Each shoulder can be treated separately, which is good for people who have to deal with a lot of stress. If you choose to sit or stand behind the client's head, place both of your hands next to each other on one shoulder (it is easier to start on the opposite side from the one from which you wish to do the rest of the treatment) and hold this position for 3 to 5 minutes. Then gently move one hand at a time, placing both hands next to each other on the other shoulder. Hold this position for 3 to 5 minutes, then slowly remove your hands and move around to the side of the client for position 10.*

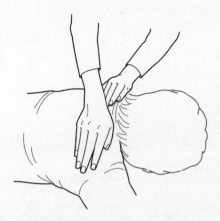

Or 9d. *To treat both shoulders at the same time while sitting or standing at the side of the client, place one hand on the left shoulder and the other hand on the right shoulder. This can involve quite a stretch, so make sure you can accomplish this comfortably; otherwise revert to 9a. Hold this position for 3 to 5 minutes, then move your hands one at a time to position 10.*

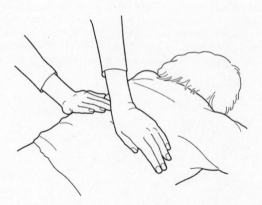

10. The back *Stand beside the client and gently without pressure place one hand in front of the other, with the palms flat against the back, midway between the shoulders and the waist. One hand should therefore be on each side of the body, and both sets of fingers should be pointing away from you. It is usual to leave a gap between your hands, where the spine is. Hold this position for 3 to 5 minutes, then move your hands one at a time to position 11.*

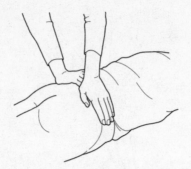

11. The waist *Gently place one hand in front of the other as before, with the palms flat against the body and the fingers pointing away from you on the person's waist, so that each side of the body is covered, leaving a small gap between the hands by the spine. Hold this position for 3 to 5 minutes, then move your hands one at a time to position 12.*

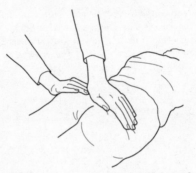

12a. The buttocks *Gently place one hand on each buttock, palms flat on the body, with each hand facing in the same direction (fingertips away from you), leaving a small gap between the hands by the spine. Hold this position for 3 to 5 minutes, then gently and slowly move your hands away and, unless you are going to treat the back of the legs and feet, move back to the client's head to start smoothing the client's aura.*

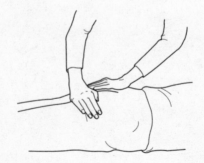

Or 12b. *Your hands can be placed gently, one on each buttock, palms flat on the body, with one hand facing to your left, and one to your right, as shown in the illustration. This can feel more comfortable for some people. Hold this position for 3 to 5 minutes, then gently and slowly move your hands away, and unless you are going to treat the back of the legs and feet, move back to the client's head to start smoothing the client's aura.*

ADDITIONAL HAND POSITIONS

Because Reiki is Divinely guided, it always flows to the areas of the physical body or energy body that needs it, and because the classic 12 hand positions enable the Reiki to flow easily and effectively into all the major chakra points, other hand positions are not really essential. However, over the years many Reiki Masters have tried other hand positions, and the commonest additional positions taught are those on the legs and feet, as shown on page 120, although these do receive Reiki when the pelvic area and buttocks are treated.

If you do use any additional hand positions such as on the legs and feet, these are usually held for only one or two minutes, but again, use your intuition, and if your hands are still experiencing a lot of sensation in a particular hand position, then continue for longer. The feet have energy zones, which correspond to all parts of the physical body, so giving Reiki to the ankles, heels, toes, and tops and soles of the feet actually sends the healing again to every organ and system within the body.

Hand Positions for Treatment on Legs and Feet

You need to stand or sit at the client's side to carry out these hand positions, although when treating the feet (especially both soles) it may be easier to stand or sit beyond the feet, as in the composite illustrations below, which show all the hand positions on the legs and feet (that is, one person in five positions, not five people).

If you decide to treat the legs and feet, then you would simply continue with the first leg position—the front of the thighs—immediately following position 8 on the front of the body, the pelvic area. You would therefore only gently awaken the client after the final position on the top of the feet, asking them to turn over. Similarly, you would continue the treatment on the back, after the buttocks, by placing your hands on the backs of the thighs, progressing down the backs of the knees, calves and ankles, and ending with the soles of the feet.

When the client is lying on his/her front

1. One hand on the back of each thigh.

2. One hand on the back of each knee.

3. One hand on the back of each shin.

4. One hand on the back of each ankle.

5. One hand on the sole of each foot (also covering the toes).

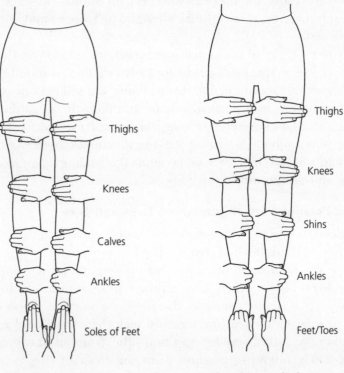

Client lying on front.   *Client lying on back.*

When the client is lying on his/her back

1. One hand on the front of each thigh.

2. One hand on the front of each knee.

3. One hand on the front of each calf.

4. One hand on the front of each ankle.

5. One hand on the top of each foot (also covering the toes).

Hand Positions for Treatment on Arms and Hands

Of course, if the client has a health problem in a particular part (or parts) of the body it makes sense to give those areas additional time, or to add a hand position if required. For example, no specific hand positions are given for the upper arms, elbows, forearms, wrists, hands or fingers, because Reiki flows down the arms, particularly when using the hand positions on the chest, shoulders and middle back—but if there is a health problem there, please treat it. It is almost impossible to treat both arms at the same time when the client is lying down, so a technique I use is as follows.

Start with one arm, and when that is completed move over to the other side of the body to treat the other arm. It does not matter which arm you start with—left or right. You can either do the arms and hands (if you have decided they need treating) immediately after hand position 5, the chest, or you can wait until you have completed the treatment on the front of the body (including the legs, if you have decided they need treating).You can then complete the front treatment by treating the arms before asking the client to turn over. Again, the illustration on page 122 shows a composite view of all three hand positions on one arm.

Left Arm

1. Place one hand on the upper arm and the other hand on the elbow. After a few minutes (not usually more than two) gently move your hands to the next hand position.

2. Place one hand on the forearm and the other hand on the wrist. After a few minutes gently move your hands to the next hand position.

3. Place one hand underneath and one on top of the client's left hand. After a few minutes gently remove your hands and move on to the next hand position—either the other arm or the solar plexus, or rouse the client and ask them to turn over.

Right Arm

1. Place one hand on the upper arm and the other hand on the elbow. After a few minutes (not usually more than two) gently move your hands to the next hand position.

2. Place one hand on the forearm and the other hand on the
    wrist. After a few minutes gently move your hands to the next
    hand position.

3. Place one hand underneath, and one on top, of the client's
    right hand. After a few minutes gently remove your hands and
    move on to the next hand position—either the other arm, or the
    solar plexus, or rouse the client and ask them to turn over.

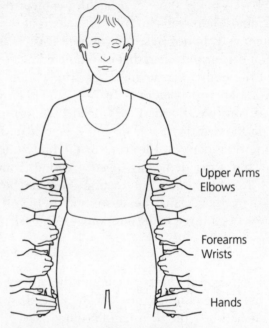

Hand positions on the arms and hands.

Basically, use the 12 hand positions of the traditional Western
full treatment as a framework, because in most cases that will be all
you need. However, if you really feel it is necessary, add to them.
Don't be afraid to be creative, because Reiki is a dynamic energy
and a living healing system, so use it in ways that feel right to you.
    Both Dr. Usui's and Dr. Hayashi's teaching manuals showed a
range of hand positions for specific illnesses, some of which used
only one hand or even just a couple of fingers. Many Reiki Masters
since then have also developed the idea that particular hand
positions can be beneficial for certain conditions. I personally
believe that because Reiki flows all around the body when a
Practitioner places his or her hands on a client, then, providing

that the Reiki continues to flow for long enough (at least an hour is preferable), every part of the physical body, as well as the mental, emotional and spiritual bodies and the whole aura, will be treated.

It is possible to give Reiki for an hour or more with the hands held in the same position—for example, with the hands on the shoulders of a person sitting in a chair—and the person will receive almost the same amount of Reiki as they would in a classic full treatment. However, this is neither as comfortable for the Practitioner nor as comforting for the client, but there may be occasions when it is the only option. But placing the hands on different parts of the body—near each of the seven chakras—does help the Reiki to flow into the body even more effectively, and it also allows a cumulative effect.

When the Reiki begins by flowing in through the crown and brow chakras, which it does in the first three hand positions, it not only flows into the head, but also flows throughout the body, beginning the process of healing, harmonizing and balancing the whole—both the physical body and the energy field. As it clears through blockages, it helps each succeeding chakra to be ready to receive even more Reiki, thus maximizing the flow. This means that it is more efficient to give a full treatment, as well as being a pleasant experience for both of you. When you try it, you will soon realize that it feels almost as good giving a treatment as receiving one, because of course you are getting some Reiki, too.

SMOOTHING THE AURA

A pleasant way to finish the whole treatment is to smooth the person's aura three times. During the treatment the Reiki has been activating and removing negative energies from the physical body into the aura, from where they can be released, and this can have a slightly agitating effect on the aura itself if the energies are just left there. Smoothing the aura down helps the energies to settle, and can detach any negative energy that is still clinging to the inner layers of the aura. It also helps the client to begin to wake up after the deep relaxation of the treatment, which could otherwise leave them feeling a bit "spaced out."

Always start at the head, and work down the body, as this echoes the natural flow of *Ki* and is soothing and calming for the client. Doing it in the other direction can have the opposite effect. Start above the crown, and keeping your hands about 30 cm (12 in) above the body, follow the contours of the body all the way down to the feet, then shake your hands downward, beyond the feet, to disperse any negative energy. Repeat this whole action three times.

AFTER THE TREATMENT

When you have smoothed down the client's aura, gently rouse them by touching their shoulder and saying their name softly. Try not to hurry the person, but if the client is still having difficulty in "coming round," gently massage their feet. When they are ready, help them to sit up or get off the therapy couch and offer them a glass of water. Also advise them to drink plenty of water for the next few days, to help the body flush out the toxins that may have been dislodged by the Reiki—but ask them to check with their doctor if they have any health problems that might be affected by greater water intake.

At this stage people often want to talk to you about what they experienced during a treatment and how they feel immediately afterward. They may also want to know what you experienced, such as where you felt any "blocks" and whether you think you have balanced those energies. At first you might be reluctant to offer such information, because it takes time and practice to build up your energetic sensitivity and intuition to help you understand what different sensations and energy patterns mean. This is because energetic sensations don't always mean the same thing. Each Practitioner may experience them and interpret them in slightly different ways, and of course there will be differences between individual clients too.

It is important to treat these issues sensibly and sensitively. You must *never* try to diagnose any illness unless you are medically qualified, but you can have an informal chat about what areas in the client's body felt warm, cool, sticky, tingly and so on. You can then ask whether they have experienced any problems there and talk in general terms about the causative issues behind illness and the messages and lessons illness offers us. You could also, perhaps, suggest that they read some of the books recommended in the Resources section to help them understand their bodies better.

It is important to realize that *you* are not responsible for their healing, *they* are, so it is not up to you to decide for them what is "wrong" with them, either on a physical or an energetic level. It is also irresponsible to frighten or offend people, so please be very careful what you say and how you say it. (It can actually be very useful to take a course in counseling, especially if you intend to offer treatments professionally.) If you have any doubts about a person's physical (or mental) condition, especially if it does not seem to be responding to Reiki treatments, then of course you should recommend gently, tactfully and as reassuringly as possible that perhaps it would be best to seek medical advice "just to be on the safe side." But please don't get too worried about all of this. Remember that you are not a "healer" but simply a channel for a Divinely guided healing energy, so trust Reiki to do its work.

Often days, or even weeks, after a Reiki treatment a person can suddenly gain insight into whatever problem area they have needed help with, because the Reiki has created an energy shift that has allowed the healing to permeate through the blockages slowly until the cause reaches the person's consciousness ready to be released.

Some people feel energized immediately after a treatment, while others feel sleepy and incredibly peaceful. If the person seems at all "spaced out," make sure you "ground" their energies before allowing them to leave. This is easily achieved by getting the client to sit with their feet flat on the floor. Place one of your hands on each of the client's feet, and visualize the energy flowing out through the soles of the feet into the ground below—hence the term "grounding." It is amazing how quickly people return to feeling normal after this simple exercise.

If they still seem a bit woozy, another good grounding exercise is to get them to stand up and then march on the spot. As they lift their left knee they should touch it with their right hand, and when they lift their right knee, touch that with their left hand. This works really well to balance the two sides of the body. If they also stamp their feet when placing them on the ground, this helps to throw the energy downward. Doing this exercise for about a minute should be quite long enough—any more is a bit exhausting.

As well as helping your client after a treatment, please don't forget yourself. You will also need a glass of water, and it is sensible to carry out some self-cleansing after every treatment. I would recommend the Dry Brushing and Reiki Shower techniques. You might also like to do some Reiki on yourself, and spend a little quiet time in contemplation or meditation.

How Many Treatments?

This is rather like asking "how long is a piece of string?" and it clearly depends upon what is being treated. For minor health problems, or to alleviate stress and encourage relaxation, one or two treatments may be enough. Major illnesses are likely to require many treatments, and afterward it might be a good idea to have a "top-up" treatment every few months to keep the energies balanced.

For very serious or chronic conditions it is generally accepted that to give four treatments, preferably on consecutive days, is an extremely valuable way to start any treatment program, because it begins the process of effectively breaking down the blockages in each of the four etheric bodies—physical, mental, emotional and spiritual—so that they are more prepared to receive and benefit from future Reiki treatments. If it is not possible to do the treatments on consecutive days, then at least two per week would be ideal. (After Second Degree you can combine hands-on treatments with distant treatments.)

Another recommendation for dealing with serious illness is to give a full treatment to the affected person every day for at least 21 days. This is obviously easier to achieve if it is a member of your own family or a friend who lives locally, but in other cases a combination of "hands-on" and distant treatments (using Second Degree techniques) can be given.

Bear in mind that in the West we are familiar with complementary health treatments lasting about an hour, so the Reiki treatment is geared to a similar time scale. However, Reiki itself is *not* geared to a specific time scale. Reiki can go on flowing—and working—for many hours, days or even weeks without stopping. We put limits on Reiki, but with Reiki there are no limits. Anything is possible. But not everything is probable.

The idea of treating someone nonstop for 24 hours a day for a week or more is not something that most of us would be willing to do. Some Reiki Masters have experimented with this (particularly Adonea, see Resources, page 303) using a number of Reiki Practitioners working in shifts in a "Reiki Marathon," usually two or three at a time, with excellent results. Now obviously a broken leg would not warrant such intensive treatment, but very serious, life-threatening illnesses could.

Even with such effort there is no guarantee that the person will recover, because we cannot know what is really best for someone—what their Soul/Higher Self knows is for that person's highest and greatest good. For many people, human life as we know it is all there is, and under such circumstances the client themselves, or their relatives and friends, might be desperate for their physical life to continue.

Their Higher Self, however, may know that they have achieved all that they came to achieve—even if they are still relatively young—and so such intense Reiki (or indeed, any number of Reiki treatments) may have a wonderfully healing effect, allowing the person to end their days in a pain-free state of tranquillity and contentment, and to make their transition peacefully.

What we must continually be aware of are the rights and autonomy of every person. Each individual has the right to seek—or to turn down—the opportunity of receiving healing. What anybody else feels about the situation is irrelevant. If someone chooses to fight an illness in any way they can, that's great, and they deserve all the support they can get. But if a person feels that there is no point, that they have reached the end and they want to give up, then that is also okay, and they still deserve all the support they can get. Reiki can help, either way. In all instances, you just need to follow your inner guidance and do what you feel is right.

WHAT IF PHYSICAL HEALING DOES NOT HAPPEN?

Reiki is not just about physical healing—it is holistic, working on many different levels, and it may be that other aspects of the person are in greater need of healing, even though we, as humans, tend to feel that physical problems should be addressed first. Another aspect I would like to mention is that not everyone wants to be healed.

Of course on a conscious level, you would expect *everybody* to choose to be healed into good health, but our motivations are often subconscious, and there may be deeper reasons why letting go of an illness, or being fully healthy, could be disadvantageous or even frightening to someone. Some people have a considerable investment in their own ill health, even if their rationale seems strange to us. Perhaps since childhood the only time they got any attention was when they were ill, or when they were sick as a child they were treated differently, or perhaps being ill means they don't have to face up to something that is going on in their lives.

Each of us is a unique individual, experiencing life in our own unique way, so it is hardly surprising that we should have complex and sometimes baffling responses to everything in our lives, including illness. Some people who try really hard to heal themselves, using all the self-help techniques available, are often puzzled and upset when their efforts are not immediately successful.

Often this is because the causative levels are very deeply buried, and need to come to the surface layer by layer to be understood, so the healing has to take time. Sometimes it is because the illness itself is the lesson that has to be learned—perhaps something that affects the mobility of the person, bringing them literally to a full stop so that they are forced to look inside and pursue insight and self-awareness.

At other times it may be because they are actually trying too hard—they are so busy "doing" things about their illness that they have forgotten how to "be." They may simply need to *acknowledge* the illness and its effects on them, reaching a level of acceptance of what it is like *in the present*, however painful or distressing that may be. In trying desperately to rid themselves of physical symptoms they may have actually blocked any real understanding of the lesson the illness was trying to teach them. Whatever happens, it is vital not to be critical of oneself, or judgmental about others, or to blame the body for not cooperating by not getting "better."

CONFIDENTIALITY AND ETHICS

Needless to say, whether you are practicing Reiki professionally or simply offering some treatments to family, friends or colleagues, any person you treat should be able to rely totally on your confidentiality, as you are in a privileged position when treating them. They may regard you as a medical professional—which you are not, unless you are medically trained—and will listen carefully to anything you say.

You may feel it necessary to advise someone to have further treatment(s) to maintain wellness—*but, as I have already said, on no account should you attempt to diagnose any illnesses*. If you feel that there is a serious problem, you should gently advise the person to seek medical help in addition to Reiki, but always in a way that will not alarm them. You may sometimes wish to encourage a client to examine their lifestyle and make positive, healthy modifications, but this should always be done with the utmost sensitivity and in a positive, helpful manner, without criticism.

It is equally important not to promise a cure, or *any* particular outcome from a treatment. The amount of healing required is decided by the person's Higher Self, and the Reiki is directed by a Higher Consciousness to those areas of greatest need—so that leaves you with very little to do other than to be a channel for the energy. Promising miracle cures is both unethical and dangerous, because you could be falsely raising hopes. Yes, miracles do sometimes happen, but no one knows when.

Another matter to think about is whether you should offer Reiki or wait to be asked. People need to know that you do Reiki; otherwise they would not know they could ask for it, so it is fine to talk about it. However, if you always offer Reiki rather than waiting to be asked, people could feel obliged to say "yes" and then you would effectively be interfering in their healing.

REIKI AS FIRST AID

Giving a full treatment is clearly not the only way to give Reiki, so don't feel constrained by the idea that you always need a therapy couch and time to do 12 hand positions. If anyone around you needs help, you have a tool available for which you only need your hands.

Many minor problems or injuries can quickly be alleviated with Reiki, such as headaches, toothaches, muscle strains, cramps, cuts and bruises and so on. Simply place your hands on the affected area and allow the Reiki to flow. In my experience most such aches and pains will ease within a few minutes and will often be completely gone within a quarter of an hour.

There is no specific amount of time for such events—just allow your inner guidance to let you know when the Reiki has stopped flowing. Usually this will mean that you no longer feel any sensation in your hands. For those people who get very little sensation anyway it may surprise you, but you will still "know" when it is right to take your hands away. Anyway, the person you are treating will probably let you know when the pain has gone.

Chapter 8

Being Creative with Your Reiki First Degree Skills

As well as being able to treat yourself, your family and friends, after a Reiki First Degree course there are plenty of other things you can do. In this chapter there are details of how to treat animals and plants, food and objects, how to send Reiki through the aura, and so on. In reality it can take a lifetime to learn the full potential of Reiki, and probably even one lifetime would not be enough, so the best advice I can give is—experiment and enjoy!

USING REIKI IN GROUPS

A Treatment with Two People

Most people consider a Reiki treatment from one person a lovely experience, but two Reiki Practitioners can treat one client, which obviously increases the amount of energy entering the recipient. Each Practitioner treats one side of the body, so their hand positions are complementary to each other, and both change hand positions at the same time, so there is no interruption in the flow of Reiki.

The following instructions should be carried out by both Practitioners as they each progress down one side of the body. Each hand position should be held for about five minutes, so the front of the body will take twenty minutes and the back of the body ten minutes. This means the treatment is completed in half the normal time, but because two people are channeling Reiki at the same time, the energy increases exponentially, so a half-hour treatment with two Practitioners is equivalent to more than an hour with one Practitioner.

Front of the Body (Left and Right Sides)

1. One hand over the eye and one hand over the ear.

2. One hand under the back of the head and one hand by the neck.

3. One hand on the upper chest and the other hand on the solar plexus.

4. One hand on the waist and the other hand on the hip bone.

Back of the Body (Left and Right Sides)

1. One hand on the shoulder and the other hand on the back (midway between shoulder and waist).

2. One hand on the waist and the other hand on one buttock.

The Benefits of Reiki Groups

Getting together with other people who do Reiki is great fun, but it also has other benefits. It can be a useful forum to discuss developments and experiences with other Practitioners, perhaps trying out new techniques or swapping tips on methods you have found useful. The more confident and experienced members can help those who are new to Reiki or who feel shy about trying it on their family or friends without getting some more practice first, so it gives them a chance to hone their skills in a friendly and nurturing environment. The more Reiki you receive, the more you heal, and the more Reiki energy will flow through you so that you can help others to heal, so Reiki groups are an ideal place to "swap" treatments with one another.

To have two, four, six or even more people treating you at once can be a delightful experience, producing an even deeper state of relaxation. (It does not have to be even numbers, but it is often easier that way.) Of course, the more people you have treating you, the less time it takes, as you simply share the hand positions among you, usually with each person working on one side of the body only. If you have lots of people you can cover all of the body and the legs, feet, arms and hands as well—and of course everyone can take turns receiving Reiki, as well as giving it.

When treating in a large group, don't feel too constrained by the traditional hand positions. It is often more comfortable to spread out a little. For example, with the head positions it would be difficult for four people to be crowded so close together all trying to treat the head at the same time.

Have one Practitioner with both their hands underneath the person's head (as in hand position 1), and then one on either side with one hand by the person's neck and the other hand by their ear. This would mean that the eyes would not be treated—but with three people treating the head area there would definitely be enough Reiki to go around. Then space people out on either side treating the body and the legs, and another at the end of the couch treating the person's feet.

If you like this idea, then why not start a Reiki group yourself? You could contact the other people who trained at the same course as you or any other Reiki Practitioners you know.

SENDING REIKI THROUGH THE AURA

There are times when it is not possible to treat someone by laying your hands on them, but Reiki can also flow through the aura, so you don't have to be right beside the person who needs help. For example, if you are at the scene of an accident, it might be inappropriate for you to offer your help directly (unless you have First Aid qualifications), but you can *intend* that Reiki should flow to the injured person(s) for their greatest and highest good. Even if they have not asked for healing, their Higher Selves will know what is needed, and will probably draw Reiki into them to help with the shock and pain.

There is no need to hold your hands out—just let the palms be open, perhaps on your lap, and simply imagine your aura expanding until it encompasses the intended recipient(s), and then mentally "switch on" the Reiki by *intending* that it should flow for the highest and greatest good.

TREATING ANIMALS

Most types of animal respond very well to Reiki, and with many you can follow a similar format of hand positions to those on humans with good effect. Clearly, though, this depends upon the size (and temperament) of the animal. There are several methods that can be used, depending upon specific circumstances:

- Placing the hands directly on the animal.

- Sending Reiki through the aura to the animal.

- Placing the hands on the cage or tank in which the animal is housed.

- Holding a small animal in your hands.

Dealing with Pets

The animals most people are keen to treat with Reiki are their pets. It seems that animals are very much more in tune with their own health and energy needs than humans, so while some will happily sit or stand for a long time to receive Reiki and keep coming back for more, others will quickly move away. Even pets who would usually sit happily to be stroked may walk off if you try to give them Reiki, and if that happens, please let them. I have seen overenthusiastic Reiki students covered in scratches or even bite marks after determined attempts to treat their pet with Reiki when the animal clearly did not want any!

Any hand positions you choose will obviously depend upon where you can reach and where the animal will allow you to touch, as well as where it is safe to touch. Also remember that Reiki will flow around the whole body, even if you can only place your hands in one position. Depending upon the size, you might try one or two hand positions on the head and two or three on either side of the body. Some animals seem to dislike Reiki being given directly onto their spine, although cats can be an exception to this.

Obviously if there is a specific injury, then that is where treatment should be concentrated, but take care not to touch any part directly that might cause the animal pain. Reiki can enter the auric field, and filter into the physical body from there, so you can hold your hands 5 to 8 cm (2 to 3 in) or more above the injury site, and the Reiki will flow in quite easily. The amount of time required for treatment will vary greatly and will depend upon the size of the animal as well as on the severity of any illness or injury.

Another way to help your pets, or other animals, is to Reiki their food and water to enhance its nutritional qualities and to offset the adverse effects of any chemicals or preservatives. This is simple to do. Hold the food or water bowl with one hand under it and one hand over it, and *intend* that Reiki should flow into the water. You can do this also with a box, packet or tin of food in your hands, intending that Reiki should flow into it—a minute is quite enough, and 30 seconds will probably do. Any homeopathic remedies or medication dispensed by a veterinarian can also be given Reiki in the same way.

Birds, Reptiles, Fish, Insects and Small Mammals

If you have a pet bird, reptile, or small mammal, they may be well used to you handling them, in which case you can just hold them between your hands and let the Reiki flow. However, if they are likely to peck, bite or scratch you, it may be more circumspect to treat them in the cage, tank or hut where they live.

Simply place your hands on or near the receptacle and *intend* that the Reiki should flow to the creature, and take your hands away when it feels appropriate to do so. Any small creatures will usually need treating for only a few minutes. Of course, if your pet needs more than one treatment, you can give it as much Reiki as you like—it is not possible to overdose on Reiki.

Farm Animals and Horses

With farm animals such as cattle, sheep, pigs, hens or geese it is often easiest to treat them through the aura from the edge of the field or beside the pen, sty or other enclosure. A horse is generally easier as they are more used to human contact, so you could place your hands in one or two positions on the head/neck, and three or four down each side of the body.

Wild Animals

It is probably best to place wild birds or other small wild animals in a cardboard box with airholes before treating them, as contact with humans can be very frightening, and the shock can even cause some to die. If you should ever need to give Reiki to an animal that might prove dangerous (for example in a zoo), or that is too nervous to let you get near it, then it is perfectly acceptable to stand a safe distance away and send the Reiki through your own aura into the auric field of the animal.

USING REIKI WITH PLANTS AND SEEDS

Seeds and plants respond extremely well to Reiki, and I have tested this many times. In one experiment I kept a houseplant alive for months without water, just by giving it Reiki each day, and I have also planted seeds in identical compost and containers and given Reiki to only half the seeds. In each case those given Reiki grew much more quickly and strongly than those that were not treated, and those planted in the Reiki half also had a 100 percent germination rate.

To give Reiki to seeds, either hold the packet between your hands or plant the seeds and hold your hands over the seed trays for a minute or two. For houseplants hold your hands on each side of the pot for about a minute or about 15 cm (6 in) away from the plant itself. If you are planting a new garden or moving plants to another border, any good gardener knows that plants become distressed and their growth is affected when moved. If you Reiki them before and after uprooting them, you should find the effects of transplantation much reduced. For any of your indoor or outdoor plants, you can Reiki their water, too, by holding your hands on or over a watering can, or when holding a hose.

USING REIKI WITH FOOD AND DRINK

One way in which Reiki can help you to achieve a healthier life is to give Reiki to everything you eat and drink. When you give Reiki to food or drink it raises its vibration so that the energy you take in is heightened. We eat food because it is full of *Ki*—life-force energy—which we need to replenish our own reserves. Adding Reiki therefore not only enhances the nutritional value of the food, but it can also help to balance the ill effects of any additives, preservatives and other chemicals, thus bringing the food into harmony with your body. However, it is still a good idea to eat organic foods whenever possible, as these are grown without the use of pesticides and contain fewer harmful chemicals.

You can Reiki your food at any stage—when you put your shopping away, when you are preparing a meal, and when you are about to eat—or all three. Before you unpack your shopping bag, place your hands on either side of it for about 30 seconds, and *intend* that Reiki should flow into the contents of the bag. When preparing a meal, or making bread or cakes, etc., assemble all your ingredients, and hold your hands near the food for about 30 seconds—or longer, if you wish—intending that Reiki should flow into it.

If the food is already prepared, either at home or if you are eating in a restaurant, you don't have to hold your hands over your food overtly—you can be discreet and hold them casually by the side of your plate or around the cup or glass for 15–30 seconds, intending that Reiki should flow into the food and drink.

I like to use Reiki as a type of blessing, and it feels good to exchange some energy with our food, because *everything* we eat was a living thing, not just meat or fish. The vegetables, fruits, nuts and seeds we eat were also alive, and they too have given up life to provide us with energy so that we may continue to live. It is therefore in line with the Reiki principle "Show appreciation and count your many blessings" to be grateful for what we eat. My invocation, as an example, is:

> Let Reiki flow into this food and drink, in grateful thanks to the Earth, the plants, the creatures and the people who have helped to bring this nourishment to me. I also give Reiki to this food to enhance its energetic quality and to bring it into harmony with my body, so that it helps my body to be vibrantly healthy and well.

USING REIKI ON INANIMATE OBJECTS

So far I have only mentioned using Reiki on living things—people, animals, plants and food—but it is possible to use Reiki on virtually anything. You may think it is incredible, but Reiki can work very well on inanimate objects like cars, computers, washing machines and vacuum cleaners—but this is not really as strange as it may sound. Everything in the Universe is energy, and all manufactured objects started out as natural materials. Once energy has been created, it cannot be destroyed, only transformed into some other state. Those natural materials may have changed *state* but they are still energy, so Reiki can still affect them.

My students and I have tried out this theory on many occasions, and successes include getting dishwashers, washing machines, vacuum cleaners, hair dryers, freezers, watches, clocks, cars and computers to work again after they had broken down. Yes, it really works, although I am not suggesting that Reiki should be used in place of proper maintenance. The principle is simple. Just place your hands on the machine that is not working, *intend* that Reiki should flow into it, and keep your hands there for a while.

I would suggest that you do so with good intentions—not out of anger that the machine has let you down, but from a feeling of appreciation for all the help the machine usually gives you. Your thoughts are energy, too, so on a purely functional level, resentful and angry thoughts would be counteracting the good the Reiki is doing.

USING REIKI ON PERSONAL PROBLEMS

As well as using Reiki on living things and inanimate objects, you can use it on more complex but less tangible things, such as situations or difficulties in your personal life, or even wider issues such as world peace (see opposite). Whatever type of problem you are having, from strained relationships with your partner or family to difficulties at work or with studying, you can use Reiki to help to permeate the situation with healing.

Simply write the situation down on paper—whether it needs a single sentence or several paragraphs—and then hold the paper between your hands, intending that Reiki should flow to the situation for the highest and greatest good. It is best to do this for at least ten minutes a day for as long as the situation exists.

Alternatively, you can visualize the situation and imagine Reiki flowing into it for the highest and greatest good, but in both cases you need to be aware that you cannot guarantee a specific outcome with Reiki. You cannot "program" Reiki to work only to change the situation to the way you want it to be, so you have to detach yourself from specific expectations about the result. This can be challenging, because it is human nature to want a particular conclusion. However, you have to trust Reiki to bring you what you need, even if that is not necessarily what you want, because that is what your Higher Self will direct it to do.

Using Reiki on World Situations

Even in the case of sending Reiki to a world situation, such as a war or famine, we don't actually know what would be best in the long term. But you can write down or picture in your mind the major aspects of that situation, and let Reiki flow into it, intending that it is for the highest and greatest good.

Even though we probably all believe that an end to all war and famine would be the greatest result, that may not necessarily be so. For example, perhaps a longer war might result in countries eventually collaborating or cooperating to produce a longer-lasting peace and stability, whereas a quicker solution might have broken down so that hostilities soon resumed. We simply don't know. However, it can only add to the ultimate good to send healing thoughts to such a situation, and the more of us who do so, the greater the chance of a good resolution, whatever or whenever that may be.

Sending Reiki Healing

Although to carry out distant healing effectively with Reiki it is more efficient to use the symbols and techniques taught at Second Degree, it is possible to send some healing at First Degree Level, although it will not be as strong. As a simile, think of distant healing at Second Degree level as being like a laser beam, where there is no diminution of strength regardless of distance, whereas at First Degree it is more like a normal flashlight beam that spreads out and loses light the farther it goes.

But don't let this put you off at giving it a try. If you want to send healing and love to people, just use photographs or write their names on a piece of paper and hold the paper or photos in your hands (or visualize them, and imagine holding their image between your hands) intending that Reiki should go to them for their greatest and highest good. Remember, though, that you cannot force healing into anyone, so if the person's Higher Self knows that it would be inappropriate for some reason, the healing will not be received and will just dissipate.

With Reiki First Degree you have a valuable tool to use for self-healing and for helping other people, animals, objects and so on, for the rest of your life. This is a tremendous gift and one that I hope you will enjoy. Many people find that Reiki 1 is sufficient for what they want to do but others want to extend their healing abilities, so in Part III we look at what possibilities Reiki Second Degree has to offer.

Part III

Developing Your Understanding—Reiki Second Degree

Chapter 9

Reiki Second
Degree Training

Second Degree Reiki is about continued self-healing and growth, but it also broadens your knowledge and healing skills to enable you to help others to heal and grow. Reiki 2 is sometimes regarded as Practitioner Level, and I would certainly recommend it for anyone wishing to practice Reiki professionally because it gives you a wide range of additional techniques to offer to potential clients.

This level is also beneficial for people who want to use Reiki more effectively on their own inner/spiritual development, so it is not simply about gaining another qualification and some additional skills in a healing technique. It is much deeper than that, because it is a significant step along your personal healing journey, and one that takes you closer to *living* Reiki—making Reiki an essential part of your daily life.

The course includes a further energy attunement (spiritual empowerment) that increases the amount of healing energy you can channel. You are taught three sacred symbols and their mantras (sacred names), each of which has its own unique healing energy, together with a range of special techniques that use one or more of the symbols. These normally include a form of distant healing that enables you to "send" a full Reiki treatment to anyone, anywhere, with the same effectiveness as if that person was with you.

Other techniques should include a special type of treatment for healing deep-seated emotional or mental problems, and healing for personal or global situations.

BEFORE THE COURSE

It is as important to choose the right Reiki Master for your Reiki Second Degree initiation as it is for Reiki 1, and most people attend a course with the same Master with whom they took First Degree. However, it is not essential to do so, and it should always be a decision based on what feels right to *you*, not what you feel obliged to do. As for Reiki 1, when deciding who to train with, ask questions, find out what the Master includes in their Reiki 2 course, and discover what their attitudes and beliefs are about Reiki—and about other things that might be important to you.

I would recommend that you follow the same suggestions for preparing for the course as in Chapter 5, but with the addition of making sure you give yourself a full self-treatment every day, preferably for a week or two beforehand if it is not already a normal part of your daily routine. Also, if you can arrange it, having a day or two before the course when you can really slow down the pace of your life, maybe meditating and spending some time in nature, would be advantageous. The same applies after the course, too, if possible.

DIFFERENT APPROACHES TO TRAINING

As you would expect, it is necessary to be attuned to Reiki 1 before attending a Second Degree course, and some Masters require you to have a gap of at least three months between First and Second Degrees, so your body has a chance to get used to the higher vibrations inaugurated by your initial attunement(s) to this healing energy.

I particularly like this slow and gentle approach, and ask my students to get plenty of practice with self-treatments (and preferably some experience with treating others) before deciding whether or not they want to take a further Reiki course. There is no time limit, so it is important to take as long as you need.

There is an increasing trend, however, for Reiki Masters to forgo this requirement and allow students to take Reiki 2 very soon after Reiki 1. The course is traditionally taught over two days, but some Masters now choose to teach it in a single day, often immediately following a one-day Reiki 1 course, so that both levels are achieved in a weekend. Naturally, the approach taken by each Master depends upon how they were trained, but unfortunately some Masters who started their Reiki journey by taking both levels in two consecutive days actually believe that Reiki does not work effectively without using the Reiki symbols—because they never got the chance to find out for themselves.

Let me reassure you. This is *not* true. There are many hundreds of thousands of Reiki First Degree students all over the world who don't choose to go on to take a Second Degree course, because they find their First Degree skills quite enough for them. So I can emphasize—Reiki *definitely* works without the symbols, although the symbols do enhance it. Also, just because you learn the symbols at Second Degree does not mean you have to use them every time you use Reiki—you can just let Reiki flow, the same as at First Degree level.

ATTUNEMENTS AT SECOND DEGREE

A Second Degree Reiki course will normally include one attunement, although occasionally some Masters perform two or three. Recent information from Japan makes it apparent that sometimes this level is split into three separate parts there, so an attunement would be given each time. However, I have always found that the single Second Degree attunement is for many students an even more profound and spiritual experience than at First Degree. Many express this as if a cloud had been lifted from them or like being reborn, so that the world looks, feels and sounds different. When observing one of my Reiki 2 classes, one of my Master students, who was very psychic, actually saw this happen during the attunement, later describing to me a misty veil being removed, leaving the students' auras lighter and clearer.

This further energy attunement also intensifies your inner healing channel, allowing far more Reiki to be channeled through—at least twice as much, and sometimes up to four times that received with First Degree, although the *quality* of the Reiki is just the same, whatever level of Reiki you have achieved. It is just the quantity that changes.

The process for a Second Degree attunement is very similar to that for First Degree, so you can expect to be asked to close your eyes throughout the procedure and to remain silent with your hands in the prayer (*Gassho*) position. Your Reiki Master will start the attunement from behind you, then they will move in front of you, and finish the process from behind you again. You will feel some gentle touching and blowing on your head and hands and at some stage may be asked to raise your hands above your head for a few moments before they are gently placed down again.

When the process is complete you should have some time to remain in a quiet, contemplative state before any further activities, and you may be given some time to yourself, for private meditation, connecting with nature, and learning the Reiki symbols.

WHAT TO EXPECT WITH A SECOND DEGREE COURSE

As we have already discussed, Masters vary in the amount of time they take to teach Second Degree, and therefore there is considerable variation in what is taught. However, there are some basics that should always be included. I think my Reiki 2 courses are fairly typical of a traditional Western approach, although some Masters might put things in a slightly different order. Also, I choose to have an evening session before the course starts, which enables me to spread the course out more to give students private study time for learning the symbols and, because I have been taught the techniques from the Japanese tradition, I include two of the most important self-cleansing methods in all my courses.

Friday

The evening session allows time for introductions, a discussion of why students have decided to take Second Degree and an outline of what the course involves. There is then a brief review of Reiki First Degree theory, including an update on the Reiki history from the Japanese tradition, which is followed by questions and answers and a guided meditation.

Saturday

We begin the morning session with an opening circle, sharing Reiki around the group, followed by demonstration and practice of the Reiki Shower and *Hatsurei-ho* from the Japanese tradition. After a short discussion of the main elements of Reiki at Second Degree—the healing practice and personal and spiritual development—the students are introduced to the three Reiki Symbols and their mantras:

1. **The Power Symbol**, sometimes called the Focus Symbol: this empowers even more Reiki to flow into whatever you are focusing on.

2. **The Harmony Symbol**, often called the Mental and Emotional Symbol: this is particularly useful for healing intellectual, psychological or emotional problems, and for creating harmony and balance.

3. **The Distant Symbol**, sometimes called the Connection Symbol: this cuts through time and space to enable you to "send" Reiki to anyone, anywhere, at any time.

There is then a discussion of some of the ways in which the symbols and their mantras can be used for treating the self, others and animals, as well as some creative uses such as empowering goals and affirmations, healing personal and global situations and Earth healing.

The afternoon session begins with a reminder about what a Reiki attunement involves and then there is a guided meditation, immediately followed by the Reiki Second Degree attunement. After this I allow my students some free time for private meditation, connecting with nature, and learning the Reiki symbols.

When we meet again later we discuss taking responsibility for our own health and well-being, and practice several different ways of using the symbols in self-treatments. We end with a short meditation and a closing circle.

Sunday

The morning begins with an opening circle and *Hatsurei-ho*, which is followed by an informal test to ensure that each student can remember the symbols accurately; this is necessary if students are to use them on each other throughout the day. There is then a discussion on the importance of energetic clearing of self and work-space in healing practice.

This is followed by demonstration and practice of Second Degree techniques for treating others, including clearing and cleansing the aura, enhancing sensitivity for scanning the body for energy distortions, beaming Reiki into the aura and carrying out a full "mental and emotional" Reiki treatment on each other using the symbols.

In the afternoon there is demonstration and practice of distant healing techniques, including sending a distant "mental and emotional" treatment and how to send healing into the past and the future. Afterward there is a question-and-answer session and a discussion of the 21-day clearing process and the Reiki practice journals required before certification. We end with a closing circle.

Other topics also come up in discussion at various times throughout the course, such as who and what can be treated, what to do if healing does not happen, what equipment is required, how many treatments are needed, confidentiality and ethics, combining Reiki with other therapies, and many of the other subjects covered in this book.

Also, although I allow plenty of time to practice the techniques during the course, I think it is essential for students to put aside time over the following few months to continue their practice of both hands-on and distant treatment techniques using the symbols. I don't issue a Second Degree certificate until I receive a copy of a student's practice journal, detailing their experiences in both.

Most traditional Reiki Masters teach a range of special techniques that use one or more of the symbols and allow time for practicing these methods, but naturally this will depend upon the length of the course. You should at least be taught the symbols, shown how to carry out some forms of distant healing, and how a hands-on treatment can be enhanced using the symbols.

Other Masters also incorporate various meditations or visualizations, as well as ways of working with spirit guides and crystals, and developing your psychic abilities, although sometimes these additional techniques are taught as a separate follow-up course, together with more advanced ways of using the Reiki symbols.

AFTER THE COURSE

In the same way as after a Reiki First Degree course, you will go through another 21-day clearing process (see Chapter 4) as your vibrationary rate is heightened and you are able to tap into a higher, wider channel of Reiki.

Reiki Second Degree operates at an even faster vibrationary rate than Reiki First Degree, and some people experience a very profound change immediately, while others notice slower changes over the following weeks and months. What is certain is that you will notice *some* changes. You may expect any one or more of a variety of effects, including enhanced color consciousness, heightened sensitivity in the crown chakra area, increased intuitive capabilities, or a feeling of greater connection with everything around you.

In many spiritual traditions it is necessary to study and meditate for many years to reach an understanding of the meaning of your own life, yet Reiki—and especially Reiki 2—awakens our sense of the connectedness with and Divinity within everyone and everything. It is important that you should honor this process as a valuable opportunity for spiritual growth. Be kind to yourself: commit yourself to do a self-treatment every day; drink between six and eight glasses of pure water each day; and try to spend some time in quiet contemplation or meditation. If possible, arrange to have at least one day afterward for gently reentering the normal world after the powerful spiritual effects of the course.

REIKI TREATMENT PRACTICE AND JOURNAL

Since one of the features of the Reiki Second Degree is that there is more to "learn" than at First Degree, it is important to put aside some time over the following weeks and months to practice using the symbols and carrying out hands-on treatments, as well as distant treatments on people and on situations. Like anything else you learn, the more you practice, the better you get, and if you use the symbols frequently in the first few weeks and months you are unlikely to ever forget them. Even if your Reiki Master does not require it, you may find it useful to keep a journal after a Reiki 2 course, detailing any of the treatments you do, and writing down any feedback you get from the friends and family on whom you practice.

As you will find in the rest of Part III, using the Reiki symbols can dramatically expand what you can do with Reiki, both for yourself and for others. There is no limit to the power and potential of the three symbols taught at Second Degree, and it would probably take you more than one lifetime to explore all the possibilities, so there is really no need to go further with Reiki unless you are particularly drawn to teach.

Chapter 10

The Reiki Second Degree Symbols

A symbol typifies, represents or recalls something such as an idea or a quality. Symbols are in common usage, and we are probably more familiar with them than we think. For example, the £ or $ signs are symbols representing money; H_2O is the chemical symbol for water; my astrological sign of Scorpio is represented by ♏; and Christianity's symbol is the familiar cross ☦.

WHAT ARE THE REIKI SYMBOLS?

There are four symbols in Usui Reiki, and each represents certain metaphysical energies. They are seen as calligraphic symbols that come from either Sanskrit, one of the world's oldest languages, or Japanese Kanji, which is the Japanese alphabet. However, they are not flat, as if drawn in ink on a piece of paper, although that may be the way they are first shown to you in a Reiki 2 course.

Their shapes are vibrational and three-dimensional, having height, width and depth. Their size is unlimited—they can be as small or as large as necessary, because they are a form of spiritual energy with its own consciousness, vibrating at a very high rate.

Of course, there are limits to the size the symbols can be drawn with your hand, which is how they are usually done. However, it is possible to *imagine* any of the symbols large enough and deep enough to encompass a whole person, a whole building or even the whole planet, or small enough to fit on a postage stamp, or inside a single cell.

Reiki symbols are transcendental in nature and they connect directly to a Higher Consciousness. Whenever a Reiki symbol is used by someone who has been attuned at Second Degree, it changes the way the Reiki energy functions. It is still Reiki, but the energy becomes empowered in different ways, depending upon which symbol (or combination of symbols) is being used. Despite their power and their spiritual nature, they are easy to use and they work automatically every time they are used—it is not necessary to be in an altered state, such as deep meditation.

The Reiki symbols are like keys that open doors to higher levels of awareness, or like buttons; whenever you "push" one, you automatically get specific action. The symbols are not the power of Reiki—but they *add* power *to* Reiki, and they are an amazing and beautiful way to connect to this higher power.

Unfortunately some people who have read about Reiki, and perhaps seen the symbols in a book or on the Internet, believe that they can use Reiki, but this is *not* the case. It is the spiritual empowerment of the attunement process that activates the symbols so that they can fulfill their intended purpose. Without the attunement, the symbols don't activate Reiki.

During an attunement, the energies of each symbol come down and enter the student's mind, body and spirit, so that afterward, whenever the student uses the symbol, the same energies they were connected to during the attunement are activated and begin flowing. Therefore, even if people do get to know about the symbols, they cannot be used for healing, or any other purpose, so it is pointless to have the symbols "out there" where people who can neither understand them nor use them can see them. Remember, Dr. Usui discovered the symbols in the sacred texts he studied, but he was not able to activate their power until after his spiritual empowerment experience on Mount Kurama.

The most usual way of drawing the symbols is with the whole hand, or with the fingers, but they can also be drawn with the eyes (in either an imaginary way or moving the eyes to follow the shape of the symbol) or even with the tongue (this one is a bit more difficult), or, when someone is really familiar with them, each symbol can be fully visualized.

Within the Reiki community there has been much debate on how necessary it is to draw the symbols correctly in order to activate them. While it is obviously important to try to draw them accurately, rather than being slapdash and careless about it—which would not respect their spiritual nature—this does not mean there is only one correct way for everyone to draw them. Indeed, we know that Mrs. Takata seems not to have drawn the symbols the same way each time, as discovered in the first meeting of Western Reiki Masters in 1982.

So variations exist between teachers, and there are certainly some differences among the symbols of the original 22 Masters she taught. She may have been guided to make slight variations in the symbols for each student, and as she did not allow her students to take notes during her courses, the Masters she taught had to rely on memory when teaching their own students, so this may account for some of the changes.

The correct way for a student to draw the symbols is the way they were shown to draw them by their Reiki Master. Everyone who has received the attunement for the symbols has symbols that work, however they are drawn, because the power of the symbols does not come from drawing them perfectly, it comes from the connections made with the energies *represented* by the symbol, during the initiation.

Differences may exist between the symbols of each student, yet each student's symbols are correct for them, and the *essence* of the symbol remains the same. It is the *intention* to use them that activates them, and brings in the specific energies associated with them. If you see Reiki symbols in a book or on the Internet, and they are different from the way you draw them, this does not mean you need to "correct" yours to follow the new version. The way your Reiki Master taught you always remains exactly right for you.

In the West we have probably become overly concerned with the symbols. From information we have received more recently from Japan, it appears that Dr. Usui began to utilize the symbols because of their specific vibrations to try to help his students feel and detect different levels of energy that existed, particularly in the human energy field.

The symbols increased the students' awareness, and helped them to develop greater abilities to discern the subtle energies that would indicate physical, mental, emotional and spiritual problems or imbalances. However, the symbols were regarded as temporary tools, which were no longer needed once a student had developed the necessary sensitivities, because with such increased awareness the energies represented by the symbols could be activated simply by intending to use them. In effect, the student would eventually "embody" the energy of the symbol.

In the 1990s some Reiki Masters began to use various other symbols within their Reiki practice and teaching. Some of these apparently came from Tibet, and others were channeled (brought into someone's consciousness by spirit guides) for use in specific ways. Although many of these symbols can be powerful aids for healing, and form the basis for other healing systems (notably Karuna Reiki® and Tera Mai™ Seichem Reiki) they have very different energetic vibrations, and are not a part of the original healing system that Dr. Usui began. The Usui Reiki Ryoho uses only the four symbols that were passed down through both the Western lineage of Usui, Hayashi and Takata and the Japanese lineage preserved through the Usui Reiki Ryoho Gakkai.

THE MANTRAS

A mantra is traditionally a word or sound that is repeated to aid concentration in meditation, particularly in Eastern spiritual traditions. Each of the Reiki symbols has a corresponding mantra, which some people mistakenly use as the symbol's name. For example, the first symbol has a three-syllable mantra, but its *name* is the Power or Focus Symbol. The second symbol, the Harmony or Mental/Emotional Symbol, also has a three-syllable mantra, while the third symbol, the Distant or Connection Symbol, has a five-syllable mantra, and the Master Symbol has a four-syllable mantra. Whenever a Reiki Symbol is used, its sacred mantra should be repeated three times, either silently, if there are other people around, or aloud if appropriate.

Each mantra works in conjunction with its related symbol, but the mantras themselves also have power, and chanting them can bring states of energy, calm, connection and bliss. I have chosen not to print the mantras in this book because they are part of the sacred traditions of Reiki, and while they are not "exclusive"—they are taught to every student who takes Second Degree—they are important, and should not be used lightly or without thought.

SACREDNESS AND THE REIKI SYMBOLS

I have refrained from including the symbols in this book for the same reasons as above. Although since the mid-1990s they have been printed in a few books, and they are now available on some sites on the Internet, I still adhere to and honor the Reiki tradition that they be kept "secret": they are only revealed to those who have taken Reiki Second Degree (or Master level in the case of the fourth symbol, explained in Chapter 19) and received the attunement that empowers them.

The "secretness" of the Reiki symbols has been misunderstood in the West, where the word "secret" is seen as shameful. In contrast, in the East the words "sacred" and "secret" are interconnected both culturally and experientially, so it would seem unnatural to people there to discuss things openly that are part of a spiritual tradition. In fact, the symbols are plainly displayed in the temple on Mount Kurama near Kyoto in Japan, and probably elsewhere in similarly sacred places—but their location clearly demonstrates that they are "special" and should be treated as such.

During a Reiki 2 course you will be shown the Reiki symbols, usually drawn on pieces of paper that you can then copy a number of times, to practice drawing them and to help you memorize them. Some Masters prefer not to have them written down, and draw them in the air instead, instructing their students to copy their actions.

Traditionally the practice papers and the original copies of the symbols are taken back by the Master at the end of the course. Often these are ceremonially burned, either before the students depart, or when the Master returns home. A few Reiki Masters nowadays give their students copies of the symbols and their mantras to keep, but ask the students not to show them to other people.

One of the reasons for taking back the copies, however, is to ensure that students are motivated to *memorize* the symbols properly, because unless they are memorized they cannot be used effectively. It may make some students feel safer having a "crib" sheet, but if you have to get out your copies of the symbols every time you want to use them, it will inhibit you too much. In the end, there is no substitute for learning.

This is where a two-day Reiki 2 course has great advantages, because there is then plenty of time to spend practicing drawing the symbols until the students feel really proficient at using them. Some Masters set a simple test on the second morning, just asking the students to take a single sheet of paper with their name on it and draw each of the three symbols together with their appropriate names and mantras, which they then hand to the Master for checking.

If after the course you do forget how to draw any of the symbols, or are just a little unsure about whether you are doing them correctly, do get in touch with your Reiki Master—it is nothing to be ashamed of, and your Reiki Master would much rather help you to recall them correctly than have the possibility of you giving up.

You are usually asked not to reveal the symbols (or their mantras) in any way to anyone other than people who have already done Reiki 2, although their nature and purpose can be discussed without violating this trust, and you can use their names—Power, Harmony and Distant. This means that you need to be careful not to allow anyone to see you drawing the symbols or hear you saying their sacred mantras. The more you practice, the easier it becomes to draw the symbols subtly, and you don't need to say the mantras aloud—you can think them, instead.

THE FIRST SYMBOL: THE POWER (OR FOCUS) SYMBOL

This symbol comes from Sanskrit, and its shape is made up of three strokes. It is probably the most versatile of the three given at Second Degree. It can be used alone or in combination with either or both of the other two symbols, usually drawn after them to bring the activating power of Reiki into their combined purposes. Its main function is to increase the power of Reiki, and to bring the energy of Reiki into the "here and now": into the present moment. In the Japanese tradition, it is referred to as the Focus Symbol, as it focuses the Reiki onto or into whatever it is drawn over.

When your body is out of balance, or you are not sufficiently "grounded," the Power (Focus) symbol works to restore an appropriate rhythm and equilibrium, to permeate things with Reiki. This will clear any negative energies and bring back the natural balance and function. It therefore helps to revitalize the body, especially the first and second chakras (root and sacral), which are linked to physical and material issues. Its main functions are empowering, cleansing and protecting.

THE SECOND SYMBOL: THE HARMONY (MENTAL/EMOTIONAL) SYMBOL

This symbol also comes from Sanskrit, and its shape is made up of nine strokes. In the West this symbol has traditionally been called the Mental and Emotional Symbol, which is a rather long and clumsy title, so the Japanese name, the Harmony Symbol, is the one I now use because it is so indicative of its actions.

It cannot be used on its own, so it is used in combination with the Power Symbol, as it has a very gentle energy and is quite subtle and more tenuous than the other symbols. Its main functions are to help to restore psychological and emotional balance, to raise sensitivity and receptivity, and to bring peace and harmony. It is particularly relevant for use with the third and fourth chakras (solar plexus and heart).

THE THIRD SYMBOL: THE DISTANT (CONNECTION) SYMBOL

This symbol is comprised of Japanese Kanji, and is made up of 22 strokes. It is perhaps the most fascinating of the symbols, because its use cuts through, or goes beyond, time and space, bringing all time into the Now, and all space into the Here. Its mantra is variously translated as "I unite with God," or "The Buddha (or Christ) in me reaches out to the Buddha (or Christ) in you to promote enlightenment and peace," which in essence means that the best part of ourselves (the Higher Self) connects, through Reiki, to the best part (the Higher Self) of others.

To use an analogy, the Distant Symbol is an energetic equivalent of a time machine, because it enables you to connect with anything, anywhere, at any time. This amazingly powerful symbol allows you to "send" healing to anyone (or anything) anywhere in the world, instantaneously, whether that is across the room, across town or across continents to the other side of the planet.

Distance is no barrier; indeed, nothing is a barrier when using this symbol, as it enables the Reiki to connect through anything— walls, rock, lead, even the Earth and outer space, to the intended recipient of the energy. All space is Here. The Reiki that is sent using the Distant Symbol loses none of its power, regardless of distance, so it is possible to "send" a complete Reiki treatment with exactly the same effectiveness as if the person (or animal) were right beside you—because energetically, they are.

The Distant Symbol can also be used to bridge time, connecting you with any time in the future or in the past, as well as in the present. All time is Now. You can therefore use it to send Reiki— including a full Reiki treatment—into the future to a point in time when you know you will need it, or to any point in the past, for example to heal the mental, emotional or spiritual effects of a past event. Again, this symbol is not used on its own, but is always used in conjunction with the Power Symbol, and sometimes also with the Harmony Symbol.

In the next few chapters you will find out how each of the three Reiki Symbols can be used, for treating yourself, others and animals, as well as many other creative uses. I hope you will have fun with them.

Chapter 11

Hands-on Treatments Using Symbols

Reiki Second Degree equips you with increased potential for carrying out Reiki treatments, but this does not mean that your Reiki 1 skills are redundant. Using symbols when treating either yourself or other people simply adds to the standard treatment, so all the hand positions remain the same, although there is an additional hand position for carrying out a specific "mental and emotional" treatment, and several other hand positions are suggested later in this chapter.

After Reiki 2 you may be keen to start practicing as a professional Reiki Practitioner, and you will find plenty of advice on how to go about that in Chapter 18. However, this and the following three chapters will give you all the information you need to actually use the three Reiki symbols, both for treatments and in other creative ways. Some of these techniques and ideas are common to many Reiki Masters. Others are unique, based on my many years of teaching and practicing Reiki, so I hope you will find them interesting, enjoyable and useful.

TREATMENTS ON OTHERS

Preparation

Just as with Reiki 1, it is probably advisable not to do full treatments on other people until after the 21-day clearing process has been completed following your attunement. Then, before starting a treatment, it is important that you should prepare yourself and the space in which the treatment is to take place, and that you put your client at ease. You will need to carry out all the suggestions in Chapter 7, including clearing and cleansing of the room and any equipment, self-cleansing and energetic protection for yourself, and the explanation to your client of what they are likely to experience.

There are some additional things you can do using the Power Symbol, to cleanse the room and the therapy couch. With the *intention* that Reiki should cleanse the room of any negative energies, go to each corner of the room in turn and, facing the corner, draw a large Power Symbol, saying its sacred mantra three times while drawing an arc with your hand from the corner toward the center of the room. When you have completed all four corners, move to the middle of the room and draw a Power Symbol above you, as if on the ceiling, and another in the direction of the floor, each time saying its sacred mantra three times.

Set up the therapy couch if you have one, and place clean pillows and blanket ready. Cleanse the couch (or other suitable place), pillows and blanket by drawing a Power Symbol over them, silently saying its sacred mantra three times with the *intention* that all this equipment be cleansed of any negative energies, and filled with Reiki.

Before you start treating your client, remember to fill your aura with Reiki, intending that the outer edge forms a protective barrier, and the Reiki within it protects you from all negativity and harm, allowing any negative energies to be released and dispersed naturally. You can then go on to sense and scan your client's aura.

SENSING AND SCANNING THE AURA

Your Second Degree attunement not only opens the chakras so that Reiki can flow even more, it also increases intuition and heightens sensitivity to subtle energies. Using the chakras in the palms of your hands, it is possible to sense where the client needs Reiki by scanning their energy field, and by scanning and healing the aura you can increase the client's ability to receive Reiki during a standard treatment. In the Japanese tradition this is called *Byosen*, and you will find details of that method in Chapter 16. However, it is possible to develop this ability quite simply.

Spend a few moments quietly tuning in to Reiki, and then sometimes it is helpful to sensitize your hands to detect energy by rubbing them together fairly vigorously for about 10 to 15 seconds—with the *intention* of sensitizing them, not just to make them warm. You can further enhance your ability to scan intuitively by drawing a Power Symbol over each hand and a Harmony Symbol in front of your Third Eye chakra, but this is optional.

Then silently ask Reiki to show you the places that need healing, and with your left (or nondominant) hand between 15 to 30 cm (6 to 12 in) above the body, start at the head and very slowly move your hand down the body, keeping your hand the same distance away.

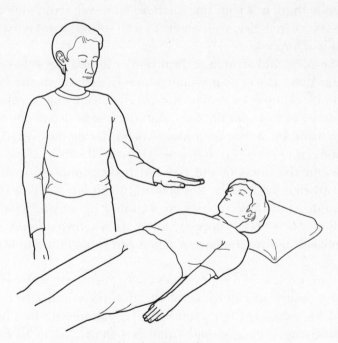

Sensing and scanning the aura.

Closing your eyes can help you to heighten the awareness in your palm so that you can recognize different types of sensation. Also it may take quite a lot of practice before you can easily identify what feelings indicate a healthy energy field, because this varies so much from person to person. Gradually, however, you will find that you will intuitively "know" what each type of sensation means. There is likely to be a "background" sensation common to most of a client's body, such as an overall warmth or very slight tingle, and often the location of a chakra is indicated by what feels like a cool breeze on your palm. Distortions or irregularities in the energy field mean that you have detected a place that needs Reiki, and you may feel these as coldness, warmth, heat, tingling, pressure, slight "stickiness," little electric shocks, pulsations or a pulling on your hand.

Your hand may also simply be guided to the right spot, and you will often "know" where the distortion is before your hand gets there. You might also find that you develop the ability to "see" or sense the energy field, and even the inside of the client's body—rather like X-ray vision—identifying areas that need special attention. These sensations and impressions may be so slight at first that you may think it is your imagination. However, trust your experience. As you practice, your ability to scan the aura and sense imbalances will improve.

When you find an area of distortion or imbalance, either make a mental note of where it is and move farther down the body to continue scanning, or deal with it directly by moving your hand up and down in that spot until you find the height where you feel the most distortion. Using both hands, palms facing downward, channel Reiki into the aura, so that Reiki can heal both that part of the aura and the areas of the physical body connected to it. Continue to channel Reiki at this spot until you feel the flow of Reiki subsiding, and then go back to scanning by moving your hand slowly down the body, stopping as before when you detect an area of imbalance, until you have scanned and healed the whole energy field.

As you work within your client's energy field, you may intuitively become aware of the cause of the distortion and any personal problems connected to it. You may also gain insight into how the problems were created and what the client can do to facilitate healing. This development may initially alarm you, if you are not used to receiving such intuitive information. However, it actually shows that you are reaching another stage in your spiritual development and growth with Reiki, so it is a good sign.

Share this information with the client only if you feel guided to do so, and then only with loving-kindness and great sensitivity, and without judgment. Always treat the client and the process with great respect, and remember, you are not a medical doctor (although some Reiki Practitioners and Masters are), so it is not permissible for you to diagnose any conditions.

A SPECIAL MENTAL AND EMOTIONAL HEALING TREATMENT

This is a very powerful treatment technique from the Western tradition that uses all three symbols, which is usually carried out immediately before a standard hands-on treatment using the 12 hand positions. If you use this method, you can then reduce the timings of the standard hand positions afterward to about three minutes (as opposed to the normal five minutes), which should still result in a treatment lasting approximately one hour. This procedure effectively floods the whole body and aura with waves of Reiki, and connects it to the Source, allowing pure love and deep healing to flow down directly into the person in a profound way.

Because this is such a spiritually intensive treatment, it is especially important to prepare yourself fully first—for example with the *Hatsurei-ho* technique and a Reiki Shower (see Chapter 15).

Another very important aspect of this treatment is that it is absolutely *crucial* to concentrate fully on the client for the duration of the "mental/emotional" part of the treatment, which lasts for between five and ten minutes. Using the symbols in this way effectively "opens up" the client's crown, heart and solar plexus chakras, in order to facilitate really deep healing. This means, however, that they are particularly susceptible to receiving your thoughts on a subconscious level, so it is imperative that you think positively rather than negatively, and that you don't let your mind wander off to think about your own concerns, problems or irritations.

The visualization technique, which is described, actually helps you to concentrate on the treatment, so it will not be as hard as it sounds. If any negative thoughts do drift into your mind, just let them go (you might like to see them drifting away inside pink bubbles). If your mind wanders off a little, just bring it back, and consciously project some positive thoughts to the client, such as "I am healthy, fit and well" or "I am calm, relaxed and all is well in my world," and then allow your concentration to return fully to your client.

ADDITIONAL HAND POSITION FOR MENTAL/ EMOTIONAL TREATMENT

This method also utilizes a new hand position, which is held for the whole of the "mental and emotional" part of the treatment. Your nondominant hand (usually your left hand) should be placed beneath the client's head (assuming the client is lying down) so that the palm of your hand cradles the base of the skull comfortably. Your dominant hand will then be free to draw the three symbols (instructions below) in front of the crown of your client's head and will then be placed directly on the crown, as shown in the illustration on page 166.

It is most comfortable to be seated slightly to one side of the client's head, so that your arms and hands can be reasonably relaxed and well supported—if you sit in an uncomfortable position it will slow the flow of Reiki because you will tense your muscles, which also tends to constrict the energy channels.

1. Before starting the treatment, ensure that both you and the client are comfortable, then ask the client to relax and close his or her eyes.

2. Sit quietly with your hands one on top of the other on your heart chakra. Reiki yourself for a few moments, breathing deeply and evenly to center yourself. Then draw the Power Symbol in front of you from the top of your head down to spiral over your solar plexus so as to clear, protect and empower you, silently saying the Power Symbol's sacred mantra three times. (Remember at all times that the Reiki symbols are sacred, and you should ensure that no one else can see the symbols being drawn or hear their mantras.)

3. Draw the Power Symbol on each of your palms, silently saying its sacred mantra to yourself three times and then scan the

client (see page 160), noting any particular areas that may require additional attention.

4. When you are ready to begin the treatment, sit down next to the client and gently slide your nondominant hand, palm upward, underneath their head—it is okay to ask them to lift their head slightly to facilitate this, as the treatment has not yet started, so they will not be disturbed by this action. Ensure that this hand position is comfortable for both you and the client.

5. With your dominant hand (usually the right) begin by drawing the Distant Symbol beside the client's crown chakra, 5–10 cm (2–4 in) away from their head (see below). Silently say its sacred mantra three times, then say the client's name three times. This establishes the link among you, Reiki and the client.

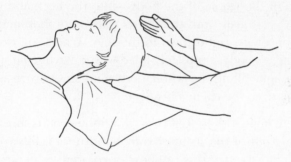

Preparing to draw the symbols.

6. Then draw the Harmony Symbol beside the client's crown chakra, silently saying its sacred mantra three times and the client's name three times. This opens the client's energy field and subconscious mind to receive all the benefits of the healing.

7. Finally draw the Power Symbol beside the client's crown chakra, silently saying its sacred mantra three times. Imagine each symbol going through the crown, brow and throat chakras and into the heart, and think, believe and *intend* that this Reiki energy is channeled with love and light for the highest and greatest good.

8. Finally, place your dominant hand (usually the right) on the client's head over the crown chakra.

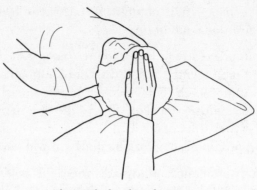

Placing the hand on the crown.

9. Now with your inner eye, visualize Reiki as soft white light flowing out of the palm of your dominant hand until it is filling the client's head, then see or sense it swirling slowly down through the whole of the body—into the neck and shoulders; down each arm; into the chest, waist and abdomen; into the hips and legs; right down to the toes. When you can visualize the client's body completely filled with soft white light, leave the white light filling the whole body, and slowly turn your attention back to the client's head.

10. Now imagine that Reiki, as a rainbow of colored light, is flowing out of the palm of your hand until it fills your client's head. Slowly take this rainbow of colored light through their whole body right down to their fingers and toes, then, leaving the rainbow light filling the whole body, allow your visioning to come back once more to their head.

11. Now visualize Reiki as brilliant, sparkling white light flowing out of your palm, becoming brighter and brighter, and imagine this brilliant white light once more flowing through the whole of your client's head and body, until every part is completely filled with brilliant, sparkling white light.

12. As soon as the client's body is filled with this brilliant white light, imagine that light spreading out of the client's body to fill the whole of their aura. Imagine it flowing into the first layer, and when that is full, see it spilling over into the second layer and then on into the third layer and then the fourth layer and

the fifth layer. Sense it spilling over into the sixth layer and then on into the seventh layer, so that the whole of the client's aura is filled with shimmering, sparkling white light.

13. Next, imagine that brilliant white light expanding still farther, until it flows out beyond your client's aura, swirling upward and outward until it fills the whole room with Reiki as sparkling white light.

14. Now visualize a strand of that Reiki as brilliant white light, coming up out of the client's solar plexus chakra or heart chakra (or both), and in your imagination take that strand of brilliant white light, still connected to your client's body, and let it lengthen until it goes through the ceiling, and then stretches up above the building, right up into the sky, and then higher and higher, through the clouds and up into the atmosphere, until it reaches the very edge of the Earth's atmosphere.

15. Now pause for a moment, and let that strand of Reiki white light gradually expand outward, see it growing and spreading out across and around the whole world, sense it meeting up with other strands of Reiki light until the whole world is covered in a fine mesh of Reiki, holding the Earth in a web of healing.

16. Then take your attention back to that narrow beam of Reiki light, and let it flow up beyond the Earth's atmosphere, farther and farther through space, past the stars, heading toward the center of the Universe, toward the Light, the Source, the All That Is. Feel it connect with the ultimate source of love and light and healing, and sense some of that love and light and healing flowing back down that strand of Reiki light. This ultimate love and healing may appear as golden light, or as any other color, but gradually it flows down the strand of Reiki light, back through space, back through the Earth's atmosphere, back down through the sky, the roof and the ceiling and into the client's body. Visualize that love, light and deep healing flooding throughout the client's body, until every part is completely filled with this beautiful, peaceful, loving energy.

17. When you intuitively sense that this process is complete, slowly take your attention back up to the connection of the strand of

Reiki light with the Source, and with a sense of gratitude and respect, gently detach the strand and begin to bring that narrow beam of Reiki back down through space, through the Earth's atmosphere, through the ceiling, until it is once more inside the client.

18. Now seal in this special healing by imagining a Power Symbol being drawn over the solar plexus chakra and/or the heart chakra, saying its sacred mantra silently three times, and *intending* that this unconditional love and deep healing be sealed into the client's body.

19. Finally, draw the Power Symbol once more beside the client's crown chakra, and silently say its sacred mantra three times, with the *intention* of closing the client's chakras and ending this part of the treatment. Closing this part of the treatment properly is *very important*. It seals in the Reiki and closes the crown chakra, which allows you to relax a little and return to a more normal level of concentration. You might like to end with a little blessing of your own, such as "I seal this treatment with love and light, and wish you joy, insight and healing through Reiki."

20. You can now begin a standard Reiki "hands-on" treatment. Since one hand is already underneath the client's head, it makes sense to start with what is normally hand position 3, so very gently slide the other hand underneath the client's head until both hands are next to each other. (You may have to move your body to facilitate this, as it will now be more comfortable if you are directly behind the client's head.) Try to do this without disturbing your client, who will probably be deeply relaxed by this stage.

21. Proceed with the rest of the hand positions—1, 2, 4, and so on—in the normal way, but you can reduce the time for each hand position to about two and a half or three minutes. (If you choose to include any additional hand positions, such as on the arms or legs, 30 seconds each will be enough after a mental/emotional treatment.) You may find it useful to draw with your hand or visualize the Power Symbol, then say the mantra three times over any areas that need special attention (for example, those that you identified during the scanning process).

Most of the time you should do all 12 hand positions, but as the mental and emotional treatment is so powerful, you may sometimes sense that the client does not need to turn over for the four back hand positions—use your intuition to decide on this—so you can spend longer on other positions.

22. End the full treatment by sealing the client's whole energy field; do this by drawing a large Power Symbol over the whole body and saying the mantra three times, *intending* to seal in the Reiki healing.

23. Then remove your hands from the recipient and place them at midchest height in the *Gassho* (prayer) position and mentally give thanks for the Reiki, bowing slightly as a mark of respect.

24. Then gently smooth the client's aura down three times, starting at the head and ending at the feet.

25. Allow the client to "come around" slowly, and give them some time to discuss their feelings or reactions to the treatment, or to ask questions. Always make sure that they are given a glass of water, and encourage them to drink about 2 liters (3½ pints) of water a day for the next three days, to help to flush any toxins out of the system that have been loosened by the Reiki. If the person seems at all "spaced out," make sure you ground them before allowing them to leave. Place one of your hands on each of their feet (on the floor) and visualize the energy being drawn down into the earth—15 to 30 seconds should be enough. If they are still not grounded, get them to stamp their feet on the floor, or to perform a cross-over balancing action, marching on the spot, and when they lift their left knee, they touch it with their right hand and the right knee with their left hand for a minute or two.

After the client has gone, sit quietly for a short while doing Reiki on yourself. I recommend that you carry out the *Hatsurei-ho* again, and/or the Reiki Shower, to cleanse and clear yourself of any unwanted energies that may have attached themselves to your energy field. Visualize or draw the Power Symbol on the walls and in the center of the room to clear and protect the room, and clear the therapy couch with a Power Symbol, too. You may also find it is a good time to carry out some Reiki projects, such as distant healing, immediately after completing such a treatment, as your Reiki energies will be flowing especially well.

ADDITIONAL HAND POSITIONS
FOR SPINE AND LIMBS

I have found the following additional hand positions very useful, either to add to a standard or mental and emotional treatment, or in cases of particular need.

The Spine

For people with back problems, this is especially good. It can be done when the client is lying on their stomach, or on their side, or even sitting or standing if they are unable to lie flat. Place one hand at the base of the spine—the coccyx—and the other hand at the top of the spine, on the neck just below the base of the skull. Hold this position for several minutes, allowing the Reiki to flow up and down the spine, between your hands. This is good energetically, too, because it allows Reiki to flow up and down the central line of energy that connects the chakras, called the *Hara* line, thus helping to clear blockages throughout the body and establish a better flow of *Ki*.

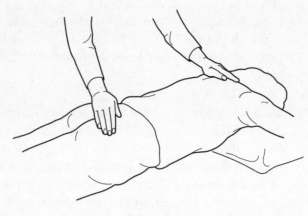

The spine.

The Arms and Hands

If someone has a problem with any part of their arm(s), this is a useful way to address it. Do the arms one at a time. Place one hand on their shoulder and your other hand on their hand, and allow the Reiki to flow up and down the arm, between your hands, for several minutes. This also helps to clear any energy blockages in the shoulder, elbow and hand chakras, to establish a clearer flow of *Ki*.

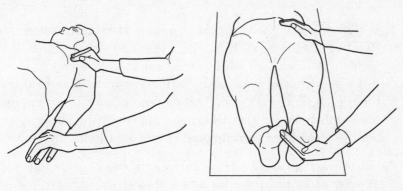

The arms and hands.   *The legs and feet.*

The Legs and Feet

If someone has a problem with any part of their leg(s) this is a useful way to address it. Do the legs one at a time. Place one hand on their hip bone, and your other hand on their foot (under the sole of the foot if possible), and allow the Reiki to flow up and down the leg between your hands, for several minutes. Again, energetically this clears minor chakras on the hips, knees, ankles and feet, allowing the *Ki* to flow more easily, which promotes good circulation and good health. It also helps to "ground" the energies at the end of a treatment.

QUICK TREATMENTS

Sometimes it is not possible to do a full treatment, so over the years I have discovered a number of ways in which you can perform a quick chakra-balancing treatment or energy boost, which can be helpful.

Chakra Clearing and Balancing

This can be done with the client either lying down or sitting upright in a chair. By working directly above or next to the chakras, in the aura, the Reiki is able to clear the chakra of blockages and balance the energies. Ask the client to close their eyes, then quietly center yourself by breathing deeply and evenly for a few moments, and *intend* that the Reiki should flow for the highest and greatest good.

1. When you feel ready, prepare yourself for the treatment by standing a little away from the client and drawing a Power Symbol over each of your palms and a large Power Symbol down the front of your body, saying its sacred mantra three times each time you do so. This empowers your whole energy field with Reiki, so that when you approach the client again both of you will be encompassed in a field of Reiki.

2. Starting at their head, draw a Power Symbol with your right (or dominant) hand in the air above their crown chakra (or in front, if they are seated) about 15–30 cm (6–12 in) away. Silently say the mantra to yourself three times and hold your hand there for approximately one minute.

3. Then move your hand to hold it above (or in front of) the brow (Third Eye) chakra, again about 15–30 cm (6–12 in) away from the head. Draw the Power Symbol in the air above (or in front of) their brow chakra, silently say the mantra three times and hold your hand there for about one minute.

4. Repeat these actions in exactly the same way for each of the remaining chakras—throat, heart, solar plexus, sacral and root—holding your hand still above (or in front of) each chakra for about one minute.

5. When you have finished, take your hand a little farther away from their body, draw a large Power Symbol in the air over (or in front of) the whole of their body and silently say the mantra three times, intending that this seals in the Reiki.

6. Then remove your hands from the recipient, place them at midchest height in the *Gassho* (prayer) position and

mentally give thanks for the Reiki, bowing slightly as a mark of respect.

7. Finally, either click your fingers, or shake your hands vigorously, to end the connection.

8. Remember to cleanse yourself afterward with Dry Brushing or the Reiki Shower.

The Reiki Sandwich

If you don't have time to do a full Reiki treatment on someone, you might find the following technique useful. It provides a quick, energy-lifting vibrational shift in the auric field. You don't have to place your hands directly on the individual, but they can remain in the auric field, just beyond the body itself, so that the client is "sandwiched" between your hands. One or two minutes in each position is usually enough, because holding your hands out can be quite tiring. Prepare yourself for doing this quick treatment in the usual way (see page 159).

1. Ask clients to either stand with their feet apart (hip width), or sit up straight on a chair with their feet flat on the floor, with their eyes closed.

2. Draw a Power Symbol on each of your palms, saying its sacred mantra silently to yourself three times. Draw a large Power Symbol in front of their body and then another at the back of their body, each time saying its sacred mantra silently three times.

3. Stand so that a client is sideways in front of you.

4. Place your hands, palms facing each other, roughly 20 cm (8 in) apart, just above the crown chakra. Hold this and each following position for about one minute (or more, if you feel this is necessary and you and the client are still reasonably comfortable).

5. Palms still facing each other, move your hands down to the Third Eye chakra, one hand 15–20 cm (6–8 in) from the front of their head and the other the same distance away from the back of their head, both palms facing toward the client.

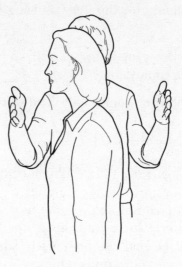

The Reiki sandwich.

6. After a minute, move your hands down to the throat chakra, one facing the front of the throat and one facing the back of the neck, the same distance away as before.

7. Next move your hands down to the heart chakra, one hand facing the center of the chest and the other hand at the same height facing the middle of the back, the same distance away as before.

8. Repeat with the solar plexus chakra, above the waist.

9. Repeat with the sacral chakra, just below the navel.

10. Repeat with the root chakra, at the base of the spine.

11. Next turn your palms to face downward, and, keeping them about the same distance away from the body as before, push your hands downward until they almost touch the floor, letting the energy flow down toward the feet to ground it. (If you cannot bend easily, then just let your palms face downward for a few seconds, and *intend* that the energy flow down toward the feet.)

12. Then turn your palms to face upward and move your hands a bit farther away from the body, say 25–30 cm (10–12 in), and slowly lift the energy as you move your hands up the whole body to the crown.

13. When your hands are above the crown chakra, briefly bring them together until your fingertips touch, and then pull them apart again, letting the palms face downward. With your hands at least 30 cm (12 in) away from the body, sweep the aura quite quickly downward as your hands move down from crown to feet.

14. Then move away from the recipient, place your hands at midchest height in the *Gassho* (prayer) position and mentally give thanks for the Reiki, bowing slightly as a mark of respect.

15. Finally, snap your fingers or clap your hands, or shake them vigorously to break the energy connection. (You can also cleanse yourself energetically with the Dry Brushing or Reiki Shower techniques afterward.)

TREATMENTS ON YOURSELF

At Second Degree level, self-healing is *still* one of the most important aspects of Reiki, not only as a part of the Spiritual Discipline of Reiki (see Chapter 17), but also as an act of self-love to give yourself a Reiki treatment every day, and a simple and sensible way to help your body to maintain good health. If you wish you can draw the Power Symbol on each hand before you start self-scanning (see below) or a self-treatment, or simply visualize it in front of you before commencing. Alternatively, you can draw the symbol, or imagine it, over each area that you are treating. Each time you use the Power Symbol, say its sacred mantra three times silently to yourself.

Self-scanning

The scanning process described earlier in this chapter can also be done on yourself and is an excellent way to get to know yourself and your energy body. If you do get any intuitive ideas, accept whatever is shown to you without judging or blaming yourself— you have simply reached the right time to increase your self-awareness in this way, and you are being shown deeper levels of yourself that need healing.

Allow the Reiki to flow into that area of your body, and your energy field, and ask Reiki also to flow into your consciousness to help you to let go of this problem area, both consciously and sub-consciously. Following this procedure regularly helps your personal and spiritual awareness and growth and increases your sensitivity, so that you become even more skilled at identifying blockages in any other people you treat.

Standard Self-treatment Enhanced with Symbols

A self-treatment can be made even more effective by using the Power Symbol. Before you start, empower your whole energy field by drawing a Power Symbol on each palm and a large Power Symbol in front of your whole body, silently saying its mantra three times each time you use it. Then, before placing your hands in each of the 12 hand positions, visualize a Power Symbol either in the air above, or directly on the body in the area that is being treated, each time silently saying its mantra three times.

Using a Mental and Emotional Treatment for Self-healing

You can considerably enhance the effectiveness of your Reiki self-treatment by carrying out a "mental and emotional" treatment, which is exactly the same as that detailed previously for using with other people. This does require considerable concentration for about five minutes or so, but you can then shorten the length of time you spend on the other hand positions, if you wish.

1. Start by sitting or lying quietly with your hands on your heart chakra, doing Reiki on yourself for a few moments. Then draw the Power Symbol from the top of your head down to your solar plexus so as to clear, protect and empower you, silently saying its sacred mantra three times. (Remember at all times that the Reiki symbols are sacred, and you should ensure that no one else can see the symbols being drawn or hear their names. It is possible to draw them very small with practice.)

2. Next, draw the Power Symbol on each of your palms, say the mantra three times, then place one hand under the back of your head so that it covers the occipital bone.

3. With the other hand, draw all three symbols over your crown chakra, starting with the Distant Symbol, saying its sacred mantra three times, then say your own name three times.

4. Then draw the Harmony Symbol, say the mantra three times and your name three times.

5. Finally, draw the Power Symbol, say the mantra three times, and imagine each symbol going through the crown, brow and throat chakras and into the heart, and think, believe and *intend* that this Reiki energy is channeled with love and light for the highest and greatest good.

6. When you have finished this, place the hand that you have used to draw the symbols on your crown chakra and begin the visualization sequence, with soft white light filling your head and body.

7. Continue with the whole of the visualization sequence (steps 9 through 17) as in the full mental/emotional treatment on pages 166–168.

8. When you have completed the visualization, seal in this special healing by drawing a Power Symbol over your solar plexus chakra and/or heart chakra. Say the mantra three times, *intending* that this unconditional love and deep healing be sealed into your body.

9. Finally, draw the Power Symbol once more over your crown chakra, and say the mantra three times, with the *intention* of closing your chakras and ending this part of the treatment. Closing this part of the treatment properly is as important for you in a self-treatment as it is when using the mental and emotional treatment with a client. It seals in the Reiki and closes the crown chakra, which means that you can then reduce your level of concentration. You can, of course, end with a statement of gratitude to Reiki for its many blessings and healing.

10. You can now continue your self-treatment in the normal way, placing your hands in each of the 12 hand positions, but you can reduce the time for each position if you wish.

The Reiki symbols are powerful and versatile, and as you have seen from this chapter, they further empower and enhance the effectiveness of any hands-on treatments, so people who have received a Reiki treatment from you before you do Second Degree may notice a difference afterward. They may remark on an increase in sensations or a deeper feeling of peacefulness. You will probably gradually notice differences too, especially in your ability to "tune in" to the areas that need the most Reiki and your capacity to interpret any sensations you feel.

In the next chapter we take a look at distant healing, where you can send one of the above treatments to anyone anywhere in the world, and it will be as effective as if you were placing your hands directly on them.

Chapter 12

Distant Healing Techniques

The techniques taught at Second Degree level enable you to send very powerful healing to anyone, anywhere, at any time, including in the past and the future. Using the Distant (Connection) Symbol allows you to connect to the person (or animal) to whom you wish to send healing, forming a "bridge" that cuts through time and space, and along which the Reiki can flow.

When you further empower the Reiki by using the Power (Focus) symbol, this means it is possible not only to send general healing— that is, simply allowing Reiki to flow to a person, animal or situation—but also to use these techniques to carry out a complete Reiki treatment on a specific person (or animal) at a distance. This will have the same effectiveness as if they were with you, receiving a hands-on treatment.

This ability to "send" powerful and effective healing into the past or into the future can even be "programed" (rather like a video recorder) to be delivered at a particular time.

There are a few points that need to be made clear before we discuss any of the specific techniques for distant healing. I use the term "send" when referring to the Reiki flowing from you to the recipient. However, apart from the initial connection, which is carried out by the Distant Symbol, it is the recipient who has to "pull" the Reiki once the connection has been made, although no conscious effort is required, as this is decided by the recipient's Higher Self. As I pointed out earlier, you cannot *force* healing onto anyone, and that includes anyone who is far away. The person or animal who is receiving the Reiki has to want it, at least on a subconscious level; otherwise the Reiki will simply come back to you.

THE ETHICS OF DISTANT HEALING

First a reminder that distant healing is something that can be sent by someone with any level of Reiki, as described on page 139, and one of the really good things about Reiki for most of us is that we have something we can use to help other people, so of course we will want to "send" healing and love to people we know are ill or in distress. Sending distant *treatments*, however, is only possible after Second Degree with the use of the Reiki Distant Symbol and is much more powerful and effective. However, there are ethical considerations for both distant healing and distant treatments, because ideally they should only be sent with the permission of the recipient.

One point to consider is that when sending healing or treatments our motives and intentions may be good, but there is also something of a controlling element in these motivations—we want someone to "get better" or "be happy." That might be *our* perception of what is for their highest and greatest good, but as I have pointed out before, we may *think* we know what that is but most of the time we probably don't.

If a person comes to you for a full hands-on Reiki treatment or asks you to put your hands on their head for some Reiki to help get rid of a headache, for example, then they obviously know what they are doing. By asking for the Reiki they are taking some responsibility for their own healing. It is equally important that the person who is to receive a distant treatment actually knows about it, other than in exceptional circumstances, such as someone in a coma. Otherwise, by sending Reiki to that person you are intruding on their personal space without permission.

Imagine if someone suddenly grabbed you by the shoulders, thrust you on a therapy couch and began giving you Reiki, without so much as a by-your-leave! You would regard that as an unwanted interference, and an infringement of your right to choose.

Well, the same is true for distant healing. You have no right to "send" a Reiki treatment to anyone, even if your motives are good and you just want to help. It has to be their choice.

Sometimes a well-meaning relative or friend of a sick person will ask you to send that person a distant Reiki treatment—but be wary. Make sure they have asked that person's permission first—unless, of course, that person is unconscious or too young or too ill to be able to make such a choice. Under those circumstances it is acceptable to attempt sending a Reiki treatment—and if the Reiki flows then their Higher Self has given permission, but if it comes back you know that it was not appropriate at that particular time.

When I say the Reiki "comes back" that might sound strange—and indeed, it can feel a bit strange. What I mean is that you make a connection with the person by using the Distant Symbol, and when you start "sending" the Reiki—or intending to allow it to flow—it reaches its destination instantaneously. This is because the Distant Symbol brings all time and space into the here and now, so it is just as if you have placed your hands on the person and the Reiki has "switched on" and started to flow into them. However, if the recipient is unwilling to receive the Reiki, it has nowhere to go, so it comes straight back across the bridge formed by the Distant Symbol and "hits" you—fairly gently, but quite definitely—in the heart chakra, solar plexus or third eye.

If this happens then close down the connection between you and the intended recipient and redirect the Reiki—you can say or think that the Reiki can flow into the planet, for instance, to heal the Earth or allow it to flow into your own body to heal you. To close down the connection, you can just draw the Power Symbol again, saying its sacred mantra three times, the person's name three times and the location once, *intending* to end the connection between you and the person concerned.

Alternatively, you can visualize the Distant Symbol as a long bridge between you and the person and visualize a Power Symbol flowing lightly across that bridge to close the connection, then gently and respectfully disconnect the end of the bridge from that person and draw it back toward you. Wherever it enters you, draw a Power Symbol over that chakra and *intend* that the process be over.

DISTANT REIKI FOR GENERAL HEALING

The first and simplest way of using the symbols to send healing and love to people—remembering the ethics set down on page 180—is to write their names on a piece of paper and hold the paper in your hands. Draw the Distant Symbol in the air over the paper, saying its sacred mantra three times, the name of the person three times and then the name of their location once (the town, area or even country will be sufficient if you don't know exactly where they are—on an energetic level, your *intention* to connect with a specific person is enough).

Then draw the Power Symbol, say its mantra three times and *intend* that Reiki should go to the person for the highest possible good—about five minutes is usually long enough. You can also use a photograph, holding it in your hands in the same way, or you can even imagine the person lying between a huge pair of hands receiving Reiki to the whole of their body or simply visualize them bathed in light. To finish, clap your hands, or shake them vigorously to end the connection.

SENDING DISTANT HEALING TO SEVERAL PEOPLE SIMULTANEOUSLY

You may sometimes wish to send distant healing on a regular basis to people—perhaps several at a time—such as friends or relatives who are ill or who are having difficulties with their studies, jobs or relationships. Again, remember that it is best to have their permission, then write all their names on a piece of paper with the towns, districts, counties or countries where they are situated, and hold this paper in your hands.

Draw the Distant Symbol in the air above the paper, say its sacred mantra three times, then say each person's name three times with their location once. Then draw the Power Symbol, say its mantra three times, say that Reiki is sent with love and light to these people for their highest and greatest good, and hold the list between your hands for between 5 and 15 minutes. (Use your intuition—you will know when the Reiki has stopped flowing.) When you finish, draw the Power Symbol again and say its mantra three times with the *intention* of ending the healing. To conclude, clap your hands, or shake them vigorously to end the connection.

Bear in mind that when sending distant healing to a number of people at the same time, it is not usually advisable to use the Harmony (Mental/Emotional) Symbol. This has the effect of opening up someone's energy field, so it should really only be used when you are concentrating specifically on one person at a time. If you need to use this symbol, you should do a full distant treatment on that person individually.

DOING A DISTANT FULL REIKI TREATMENT

Using this technique enables you to send a full Reiki treatment with exactly the same effect as if you were carrying out a hands-on treatment on that person or animal. It is very simple to do and takes much less time than a hands-on treatment, but it does require a considerable amount of concentration, so you need to be somewhere quiet where you will not be disturbed for 20 minutes or so before starting.

Because this treatment works in the same way as if the person was with you, it is particularly important that you should have their permission before sending the treatment, and ideally you should arrange a convenient time when that person can be sitting comfortably or lying down somewhere quiet where they will not be disturbed for at least three quarters of an hour. (This amount of time is to allow them some relaxation after the treatment.)

While Reiki always works for the highest and greatest good, it is probably sensible to avoid sending a full treatment when you don't know what the person is doing, as Reiki often makes people feel very relaxed or even a bit drowsy. If they were driving or operating machinery, for example, this could potentially make it more difficult for them, so in situations where you are not sure what they are doing you can "program" the treatment for when they are asleep at night—more details later in this chapter.

Despite this caution, note that I know of several instances similar to the following: a distant treatment was sent at an agreed time, but the person who was due to receive it had to deal with an emergency and was up a ladder, fixing a roof. Obviously, at that point receiving

Reiki might have been inappropriate, so the Reiki "waited" until
the person had finished and was putting the ladder back in his
garage, at which point he actually felt the Reiki "descend" and was
able to go into his house quickly and sit in a comfortable chair to
receive it properly.

USING A "CORRESPONDENCE"

You can use a "correspondence"—something you use to represent
the person and on which you can place your hands during the
treatment "as if " they were on the person. This could be your own
knee and thigh or a pillow or even a teddy bear or some other
cuddly toy. This works because everything is energy and therefore
everything is connected, so when you use an object to represent
(correspond to) something else your intention transmutes the
energy esoterically, so that for a period of time the correspondence
"is" the body of someone else. (Yes, I know it sounds a bit weird,
but it does work!)

You don't have to use an object as a correspondence. Photographs and names written on pieces of paper also act as corre-
spondences, as do images that you visualize. When visualizing a
person you can imagine them to be life-size or the same size as a
pillow or teddy bear, or really small so that they would fit into your
hand. You could then use visualization to imagine your hands in
different positions on the body—or you could visualize the person
held between huge hands, so that all parts of their body would be
receiving Reiki at the same time.

One word of caution: when using the Distant Symbol you create
a really powerful connection; when they are receiving a distant
treatment many people who are energetically quite sensitive actually feel as though the Practitioner's hands are on their body, and
they can feel when the hands move to be placed elsewhere. While
this is excellent, it does mean that you must be as careful when
doing a distant treatment as when doing a hands-on treatment, so
make sure all your hand movements are gentle.

The main caution in this case, however, is about imagining the
person turning over (or physically turning over whatever you are
using as a correspondence) to have their back treated. Please do

this *very slowly and gently* as the energetically sensitive person can become very disturbed by this, and can sometimes feel the need to actually turn over, so you must give them time to do this. I know of people who have fallen off a sofa or out of bed in the middle of receiving a distant treatment when the Practitioner "flipped" them too quickly onto their stomachs—even though they were many miles apart at the time!

DISTANT TREATMENT METHODS

A Standard Distant Treatment

1. Prepare yourself for doing the treatment. You should sit somewhere comfortable and quiet, where you will not be disturbed—switch the telephone off, ask the family to leave you alone for half an hour, and so on. You might choose to light some incense or burn some aromatherapy oil and have some gentle music on in the background if you wish. Spend a few minutes meditating—doing the *Hatsurei-ho* is a good way to prepare yourself, as it will also cleanse your energy field.

2. Picture the person to whom you wish to send the Distant Reiki treatment. You can use a photograph or write their name and address on a piece of paper, or you can just visualize them. You can also use a "correspondence"—something that you can use to represent the person, as described above. Just imagine that whatever you are using as a correspondence is the person, so spend a few moments deciding which part represents their head, which represents their body, legs, and so on.

3. Draw the Distant Symbol over the photograph, paper or body of the correspondence, say its mantra three times, the name of the person three times and their location once (either their whole address or just the town, area or country they are in, if you don't know exactly where they are). Just imagine the Distant Symbol going out like a huge bridge between you and the person to whom you are sending a distant treatment.

4. Then draw the Power Symbol over the photograph, paper or body of the correspondence, say its mantra three times, the name of the person once and their location once. Imagine a

large Power Symbol over the body of the person, then let it descend so that the person is completely encompassed by the symbol, enabling its healing energy to flow throughout the person during the treatment.

5. Then say that this Reiki is sent with love and light, for the highest and greatest good. (You may also mention any specific parts of the body or illnesses or situations that you know need special attention and ask that they receive healing if this is possible at this time, but it will be the person's Higher Self who decides how to use the energy, so try not to have specific expectations—that is, it is important to take our ego out of the healing process.)

6. You can then carry out a standard treatment by placing your hands as if they were in each of the 12 standard hand positions, either actually on the correspondence—a pillow is especially good, because it is long enough to fit your hands on—or in the air above a photograph, etc. Start with hand position one over the eyes, and hold that, then each following hand position for 3 minutes for those on the head and body and for 1 minute on any other hand positions you choose to do, such as the arms, legs and feet.

7. When you have finished, close the whole treatment by smoothing down the person's aura with your hands (in the air or over the pillow, etc.), then draw a Power Symbol over the whole of their body (starting at the head), again saying its sacred mantra three times, with the *intention* of closing the person's chakras and ending the treatment.

8. I like to end with my hands in the prayer position (*Gassho*), to show respect and mentally thank the Reiki, and then clap my hands together firmly (usually three times) to break the energy connection. Afterward I spend a few minutes in quiet contemplation, and then carry out some self-cleansing—either the Reiki Shower or Dry Brushing technique or the whole of *Hatsurei-ho*.

A Mental/Emotional Distant Treatment

This is an even more powerful way of doing a distant treatment. It works deeply on the psychological or emotional causative levels, helping blockages to rise to the surface to be healed and released, so this is the method I usually use. The visualization helps to keep your mind really focused on the person receiving the treatment, which is essential, as their chakras are opened by the Harmony Symbol in order that they can receive the maximum amount of Reiki. Just as in the hands-on treatment of the same name (see previous chapter), it is important to project only positive thoughts during the sending of this treatment.

1. Carry out the same preparations as in steps 1 and 2 of the standard distant treatment on page 185.

2. When you are ready, place your nondominant hand underneath the photograph, paper or correspondence (whichever part you have decided represents the head), and draw the Distant Symbol in the air above the photograph, paper or correspondence, say its sacred mantra three times followed by the name of the person three times and their location once, and direct its energy to whatever represents the crown of the recipient.

3. Draw the Harmony Symbol, say the mantra three times and the name of the person three times and direct its energy to the crown of the person.

4. Draw the Power Symbol, say the mantra three times, directing its energy to the crown of the person, and *intend* and say that this powerful Reiki healing is sent with love and light, for the highest and greatest good of (name of person).

5. Carry out a full mental and emotional treatment on the person, using the visualization in steps 9–17 on pages 166–168 in chapter 11, remembering to maintain your full attention on the person. When this has been completed, draw a Power Symbol and say the mantra three times over whatever represents the person's crown chakra, *intending* that the mental and emotional part of the treatment has ended. Remember that it is really important to end this part of the treatment properly. You can then relax your concentration for the next part of the treatment.

6. Then carry out a shortened standard distant treatment, as in step 6 on page 186 reducing the timing of the hand positions on the head and body to 1 or 2 minutes each. (The shortened standard treatment can even be omitted if necessary, although it is clearly better to include it whenever possible.)

7. Finally smooth the aura, close the treatment with the Power Symbol, and carry out your own cleansing as in step 8 on page 186.

PROGRAMING THE TREATMENT FOR A FUTURE TIME

If you are unable to agree on a particular time, or if you have another commitment at the time that is suitable to a potential recipient, then it is possible to "program" the treatment to go to them either at a specific time arranged between you or while they are asleep, rather like setting a video recorder to record a television program at a particular time.

To do this, follow the instructions on page 185 for carrying out a standard distant treatment until you have completed number 5, and then say "This Reiki is to be received by (name of person) at (time agreed), or "when they are asleep tonight," or even "when it will be most beneficial." You can also preprogram a mental/emotional distant treatment in exactly the same way.

PROGRAMING FOR REPEAT-HEALING TREATMENTS

If there is a requirement to send a person lots of treatments—say, for example, someone needs 21 consecutive treatments to help with some chronic or life-threatening condition—it will take you about 15 to 20 minutes a day to carry these out. However, there may be times when you have a few daily treatments to do on other people, or perhaps you have some serious commitments and are unsure of being available to carry out the distant treatments at the right time.

It is possible to "program" a treatment to be received regularly at the same time each day, without your having to sit there doing it every time—again, rather like programing a video recorder to record the same television program daily at the same time. Remember, the Distant Symbol cuts through time and space, so this is no problem.

Carry out either the standard distant treatment or the mental/emotional distant treatment in exactly the same way as in the above sections, but when you reach step 5, add the following instruction: "This Reiki is to be received by (name of person) at (time agreed) or "when they are asleep (today or tonight) and for the following six days (or nights)." Then, after one week, you can either get back to doing the distant treatment on a daily basis, or if the same conditions exist for you, you can reprogram the treatment for another seven days.

If someone is very ill or perhaps is unconscious or experiencing some other dangerous health crisis, a useful tip is to program a treatment to go to them every hour or every two hours. For this you would carry out either of the above distant treatment instructions up to number 5, and then say "Let a full Reiki treatment flow to (name of person) every hour (or every two hours) for the next 48 hours." Again, after the two days you can review the situation and see whether you need to reprogram it in the same way or reduce the number of treatments, and so on.

How to Send Treatments to Several People Simultaneously

Whenever possible it is obviously best to put aside the time needed for an individual distant treatment, but when time is short, or if you have a number of close friends or relatives who need regular distant treatments, this can involve a considerable time commitment on your part, as each treatment (particularly the mental/emotional treatment) can take 20 minutes or more. It is therefore possible to send a full distant Reiki treatment to a number of people at the same time—but *not* the mental/emotional treatment, as this really does require all your attention to be on one individual.

You can use a single correspondence, such as a pillow, on which to place your hands, and then have photographs of each person nearby or their names and addresses on pieces of paper. I would suggest that you limit this to three people. (You can visualize them but it is difficult to keep all their images in your mind.)

Draw the Distant Symbol over one photograph (or name), saying its mantra three times, the name of that person three times and their location once. Then over the same photograph (or name) draw the Power Symbol and say the mantra three times.

Repeat this process with each of the other photographs (or names), then place your hands over the correspondence you are going to use. Draw the Distant Symbol again, say (aloud) "This pillow (or whatever else you are using) represents each of the following people (say each name and location three times—for example, Joe Bloggs in London) so that a complete Reiki treatment now flows to all of the people I have named for their highest and greatest good."

Then draw the Power Symbol over the correspondence, say the mantra three times and commence the treatment by placing your hands in position 1 for a couple of minutes, then moving them gently to position 2 and so on. Finish the treatment by smoothing the aura three times (from head to feet). Finally, draw the Power Symbol again over the pillow and once over each photograph/name, say the mantra three times for each and *intend* that the distant treatment be over. To conclude, clap your hands three times or shake them vigorously to end the connection, then mentally thank the Reiki and finish by carrying out some self-cleansing.

Note that I am *not* suggesting the use of the Harmony Symbol in this multiple treatment, but as your *intention* is for each person to receive a full Reiki treatment for their highest and greatest good, they will all receive whatever Reiki they need individually. As I said earlier, if you feel that the person would benefit greatly from a mental/emotional treatment, you need to do a separate treatment on that person.

We have been concentrating on distant healing for people in this chapter, but there are some other ways to use distant healing techniques, for example for personal problems and world situations. These and other creative ideas are given in the next two chapters.

Chapter 13

Other Uses
for the Reiki Symbols

There are many things that you can do to enhance your life when using the Reiki Symbols in addition to treating yourself and other people. The symbols are so versatile that the list is almost endless, but I have written down some of the most useful ideas in this and the next chapter. There are techniques for using the symbols around the home and at work; using them for clearing, cleansing and creating sacred space; using them for healing bad habits and other situations, and more. I hope you have fun trying them out.

USING SYMBOLS WHEN TREATING ANIMALS, BIRDS, REPTILES, FISH OR INSECTS

With the Second Degree symbols, you will find it even easier to treat animals, birds, reptiles, fish or insects. You can use the Distant Symbol to connect to any type of creature anywhere and at any time, and the Power Symbol to bring the Reiki powerfully to it; you can do this from any distance away.

Another way to help animals is to draw the Power Symbol over their food and water (saying the mantra three times) to enhance its nutritional qualities and to offset any adverse effects of any chemicals or preservatives. Any homeopathic remedies or medication dispensed by a veterinarian can be treated in the same way.

Using the Symbols with Plants and Seeds

When you walk past any of your houseplants, occasionally draw the Power Symbol over them, saying its mantra three times and intending that the Reiki flow for the plants' highest good. The same applies to plants in your garden, yard or patio; to the crops in your allotment or fields; and to seeds or cuttings. You can also treat plants using the Distant Symbol before the Power Symbol, if you are away on holiday, for instance.

Using the Symbols with Inanimate Objects

The symbols, especially the Power Symbol, can be used to enhance any Reiki you might give to machinery or equipment that is not working. Either draw the Power Symbol in front of or over the machine, or draw the Power Symbol over each of your palms before placing your hands on it. For an object far away, simply connect with it using the Distant Symbol, saying its mantra three times and the name of the object three times. Then use the Power Symbol, say the mantra three times and *intend* that Reiki should flow into the object for the highest possible good.

Using the Symbols with Food and Drink

The Power Symbol and its mantra can be used over all food and drink, including the food on your plate and all the ingredients when you are cooking.

Using the Symbols on Personal Problems and Situations

Whatever kind of problems you are having, from strained relationships with your partner or family to difficulties at work or with studying, you can use Reiki to help to permeate the situation with healing.

1. First, write down the details of any problem area you are working on and hold the paper between your hands. Examples could be "Allow Reiki to flow into the situation of my relationships, for the highest and greatest good" or "Let Reiki flow into the situation of my money issues, for my highest and greatest good."

2. Then draw the Distant Symbol over the paper, silently saying its mantra three times, and intending that the Reiki connect with the situation.

3. Next draw the Harmony Symbol over the paper, and say its mantra three times, asking that Reiki flow to harmonize and heal the situation in whatever way is for your highest and greatest good.

4. Then draw the Power Symbol over the paper and say its mantra three times, intending that Reiki flow into this situation for the highest and greatest good.

5. Maintain this position for 5 to 10 minutes, and when you have finished, thank Reiki for its help, draw another Power Symbol, and say its mantra three times over the paper, intending that the healing is sealed in, and the treatment is over.

6. Do this each day, and continue to work on this situation until some resolution to the situation appears.

EMPOWERING GOALS WITH REIKI SYMBOLS

You can use a similar method for working on your goals and dreams with Reiki. Write down what you really want—a new job, a loving relationship, a cottage in the country, a trip to Disneyland— on a piece of paper; be as specific as possible. Write down *all* the aspects of what you are seeking, so if you want a cottage in the country, put down how many bedrooms and bathrooms you want, what kind of kitchen, whether you want central heating or open fires, a small garden or acres of farmland, and so on.

Then draw the Distant Symbol over the paper and say its

mantra three times. Then draw the Harmony Symbol and say its mantra three times. Finally draw the Power Symbol. Say its mantra three times, then hold this piece of paper in your hands and *intend* that Reiki should flow into that goal for the highest and greatest good. Give it Reiki for at least ten minutes a day until you achieve what you want.

But beware. Be sure that you *really* want it before you ask for it, because if your goal is in harmony with your highest good, you will achieve it. However, your highest good can sometimes be served by going through negative experiences, as well as positive ones, so sometimes the outcome might not be as rosy as you expected. For example, lots of people dream of winning millions of pounds or dollars, but when they do they find it a dreadful responsibility, causing friction in the family and huge changes in their lifestyle that don't make them happy after all. This might be because their friends don't want to be around them so much, since they feel uncomfortable about not being able to keep up with their spending power. But those are valid life lessons too. See what I mean?

It is also necessary to think about whether what you are asking for is ethical. For example, if you have a specific house in mind but it is not actually for sale and there are people already living there, there are any number of reasons—pleasant and unpleasant—why the current owners might have to put it on the market. Much better to describe the type of home and location you are seeking, rather than a specific property.

Another ethical question is about relationships. You may have a specific person in mind with whom you would like to develop a close, intimate relationship, but even if that person is free and single, it is *not* appropriate to work with Reiki in this way. It would be an infringement of that person's rights and would be interfering with their emotional choices.

EMPOWERING AFFIRMATIONS WITH REIKI SYMBOLS

If you are working with affirmations—positive statements that can help to reprogram your thinking—these can be made even more effective by writing them down, drawing the Reiki symbols over them, holding the paper in your hands, then saying them over and over to yourself while giving them Reiki. (You can use all three symbols for this, together with their mantras, in the usual order: Distant, Harmony and Power.)

This can be a really powerful method for change, so make sure that your affirmations are always really positive, with an intention for your highest and greatest good, and that they are fully in the present. So, for example, use "I have a wonderful, loving relationship with a man/woman who loves me" even if this is not the case right now, rather than "I will have ..." or "I would like ...," and "My body is healthy and full of vitality" rather than "I am not ill anymore."

This is important, because what we think, say and feel *now*, at this moment in time, is what is creating our future. In that context our minds and bodies see no difference between "real" or "imagined" reality. For example, some research in Japan (reported in the *Kyushi Journal of Medical Science* in 1962) found that blindfolded children who were told that poison ivy was being brushed against their arms produced swelling, redness and itching on their skin, even when the plant used was perfectly harmless. Their beliefs produced what they expected would happen. When we use affirmations we are affirming what we want to be true and feeling and acting upon it as if it were true. This creates the right positive climate to manifest and make it real for ourselves.

Try the power of words for yourself. To demonstrate it more dramatically, you can start with a negative statement, so say aloud "I feel sad" at least ten times; your body will start to droop and your voice will become quieter and sadder. But then immediately afterward use a positive affirmation by saying "I am happy" between 10 and 20 times, and your body will begin to straighten up again, your voice will lift, and eventually it will be hard to suppress a smile!

Because Reiki will always work for your highest and greatest good, it will help you to achieve your ideal, but it may first produce results that force you to face up to the blocks that are currently preventing you from having what you want. For instance, if you are desperate to form a loving relationship this might be because you don't feel you are a whole person without a partner. This could indicate that you need to work on your self-esteem and ability to love yourself, so it is likely that these issues would arise first. So you get what you need, rather than what you want—but at least you will be a step closer.

USING SYMBOLS TO HEAL UNWANTED HABITS OR ADDICTIONS

The Harmony Symbol can be used to help you change or eliminate habits or addictions that are no longer useful to you, such as smoking cigarettes, drinking alcohol, taking nonprescription drugs or even overeating. However, it is important that you should actually *want* to give up the habit that you are working on, because you recognize the benefits to yourself and acknowledge those benefits as being more advantageous than whatever it is that the habit gives you. Reiki can be of considerable assistance, but it cannot force you to do something you don't want to do, or something you are only doing to please someone else.

The Harmony Symbol works on the psychological and emotional causes underlying things, and each of the above-mentioned habits has its root in at least one, and probably both, of these potential causative issues. Using the Harmony Symbol will help to bring the causative issues to the surface—such as rejection, fear, anxiety, self-loathing, the need for affection, and so on—so that they can be examined and healed.

Such self-realizations can, of course, be very uncomfortable, so if you don't really want to tackle the problem you will simply push it back under the surface and nothing will be achieved. But if you really do want to work on the problem, Reiki can help you to change to better, healthier habits as well as help you to heal and let go of whatever issues have been underlying your habit. It can also allow you to let go of the problem enough to feel a sense of gratitude for the lessons it has taught you, because every experience has value in the insights it offers and its contribution to who you are right now.

Write your name on a piece of paper, together with a suitably positive statement such as "I am now choosing a healthier lifestyle, so I choose to heal and let go of my need to smoke/drink alcohol/ overeat/take drugs." In the air above the paper draw a Harmony

Symbol, silently saying its mantra three times and repeating aloud three times the statement you have written, then draw a Power Symbol and say its mantra three times. Hold the paper between your hands, treating it with Reiki for 15 to 20 minutes a day. Continue to do this until you feel that you have really let go of this unwanted habit.

CLEANSING AND CREATING SACRED SPACE

Any space can become contaminated with negative energy, or negative energy can simply collect and stagnate in corners. The more you become involved in your spiritual path, the more important it is not to be surrounded by negativity, so use Reiki everywhere, all the time, to create positive space around you.

The simplest and easiest way of clearing negative energy from your surroundings is to place Power Symbols all around you—in all the corners and sides of any room, plus the ceiling and floor. Draw the Power Symbol (as large as possible, if no one is watching; otherwise draw it discreetly) and say its mantra three times in each place. *Intend* that the Reiki should clear and cleanse the room and seal it in light, making it a sacred space. This is good not only for any room in your home, but also in your workplace, in hotel bedrooms, in hospital wards or anywhere else you are staying.

You can cleanse just about anything with Reiki, using the Power Symbol and *intending* that the Reiki cleanse whatever you are directing it at. You can try it on your bed, your clothes, your car— in fact anything in your life that might attract or hold negative energy. You can also use the Power Symbol to cleanse yourself if you have been somewhere that you feel was energetically rather negative, for example after visiting people in the hospital or after attending a funeral.

Draw a Power Symbol (discreetly) in the air above your crown chakra, saying its mantra three times, and intending that the Reiki cleanse your whole energy field. Imagine the Power Symbol growing and extending until it fills your aura, then imagine it moving downward toward the ground, taking with it any negative energy until the negativity flows into the earth with the

Reiki, which will heal it and transmute it so that it is useful energy for the planet.

USING THE SYMBOLS FOR PROTECTION

The Power Symbol can be used for protection, and because Reiki works on all levels, the protection it provides is also on all levels and includes protection from physical harm, verbal and emotional confrontations and psychic attack. It can be used to protect your car, your home, your children or anything else you value, and you can use it to protect yourself and your family when you are traveling, too.

There are a variety of ways of using Reiki for protection, and I have given some of the most popular ones below. Be inventive—you may think of other ways.

Self-protection

This is best repeated on a daily basis, and again in any situations that call for it.

- *Either* draw a large Power Symbol in front of you and step into it, silently saying its sacred mantra three times, and imagining it encompassing you and intending that it form a protective barrier around you.

- *Or* draw a Power Symbol in front of you, and on each side of you, and imagine drawing one behind you, saying its mantra three times, and intending that it form a protective shield around you. You can also add a Power Symbol over your head and beneath your feet, if you like.

Your Car, Home or Other Objects You Care About

This is best repeated on a weekly basis. Either physically draw, or imagine drawing, a large Power Symbol over the object, saying its mantra three times, then imagine the Power Symbol expanding until it covers the object above, below and on all sides. *Intend* that the Power Symbol protect that object for as long as is necessary. (If you are away from the object, use the Distant Symbol to connect with it first.)

When Traveling

If you know your destination, discreetly draw a Distant Symbol, thinking its mantra three times, and imagine it forming a bridge of light connecting you with your destination. Then imagine a large Power Symbol over your car or the bus, train, ship or aircraft you are traveling in, say its mantra three times and imagine the Power Symbol spreading until it covers your means of transport above, below and on all sides. *Intend* that the Power Symbol protect all the occupants of that means of transport for the duration of the journey. You can then imagine a Power Symbol traveling ahead, clearing the way for you along the bridge of light formed by the Distant Symbol.

For Children

There may be occasions when your children are not with you and you sense that they may need protection. You can connect with them using the Distant Symbol, and then imagine a large Power Symbol encompassing them, *intending* that it protect them for their highest and greatest good.

Be sensitive to the fact that this is actually a controlling and potentially intrusive thing to do—you are deciding what is best for them, because you love them and want them to be safe. This is natural enough, but their highest good may not be best served by being so protected—children need challenges to help their personal and social development. If they are old enough to understand, I think it is always best to ask their permission first. Then, if they want Reiki protection, they are choosing it rather than having it thrust upon them.

USING THE SYMBOLS FOR MOTIVATION, MEMORY AND SELF-GROWTH

The symbols can be used to enhance various aspects of mental performance, such as the following:

For Self-motivation

Draw a Power Symbol over your forehead, saying its mantra three times, *intending* to increase your motivation in general or for specific tasks.

To Help Your Memory

Either draw a Power Symbol over the top of your head or the Harmony and Power Symbols on your crown and brow chakras, saying their mantras three times and *intending* that Reiki should help you to remember whatever it is you need to remember.

To Help You Learn Things

This can be used, for example, for exams or interviews. Use the Harmony and Power Symbols on your crown and third eye chakras and also draw them over the passages, chapters or information you need to learn, silently saying their mantras three times and *intending* that Reiki help you to learn.

For Self-growth and Increased Understanding

Draw the Harmony Symbol, followed by the Power Symbol, on both palms, then hold your head with both hands either on your brow and the back of your head or on both sides. Imagine the symbols entering your head, and as you silently say the symbols' sacred mantras *intend* that the Reiki help you with your self-growth and understanding.

For Achieving Goals, Dreams and Ambitions

Draw the Harmony Symbol followed by the Power Symbol on both hands, then hold your head with one hand on your forehead and the other hand on the back of your head, saying their sacred mantra three times and *intending* that Reiki help you to achieve your goals, dreams and ambitions.

USING THE SYMBOLS WITH EMOTIONAL ISSUES

The Harmony Symbol, when used together with the Distant and Power Symbols, is the most useful for helping you to improve all kinds of relationships, from family to friendships and business contacts. Of course, you cannot determine the outcome because the Reiki will still be acting for your highest and greatest good. But generally you will find that there is some improvement, as the people involved will be aware, on an energetic level (and through their Soul/Higher Self), that you are trying to create greater harmony for the good of you all.

For Relationships of All Kinds

This can be repeated as often as necessary—even on a daily basis, until the relationship shows signs of developing greater harmony. It is helpful to imagine the pairings or groups of people (for example, you and your partner; or you and your work colleagues) all together, perhaps sitting on or around a sofa.

Draw the Distant Symbol to connect to the group, the Harmony Symbol to bring peace and harmony and the Power Symbol to bring healing energy to the situation, saying their mantras three times and a description of the group once (for example, my wife and me; or Bill, Wendy, Jean and myself at work). Then imagine the Harmony Symbol as if it is hovering above the group and watch it gently descend until it encompasses the whole group. *Intend* that it bring its peaceful, harmonious energies to the group for the greatest and highest good.

Hold this image for about five minutes—you can turn it into a visualization if you want, seeing the people involved getting along better and perhaps ending with a hug. Then draw the Power Symbol, say its mantra three times and *intend* that the healing be complete. Then clap your hands or shake them vigorously to break the connection.

For Meetings of All Kinds

Do the same as above, but perhaps imagine the appropriate group of people sitting around a table. If you don't know all their names or don't know what they look like it does not matter, just specify "all the people at my interview" or "all the people at the Council meeting," etc. As you are using the Distant Symbol you can also specify the time of the meeting or interview, and when you hold the image of the group you can perhaps "see" the meeting ending with everyone smiling and shaking hands.

For Emotional Issues of All Kinds

This can be repeated as often as necessary. To deal with nervousness, fear, depression, anger, sadness, restlessness, impatience, stress or tiredness, draw or imagine a large Harmony Symbol over your crown chakra, then visualize the symbol expanding until it encompasses the whole of you. Say its mantra three times and ask and *intend* that it bring its gentle, healing, peaceful and restorative energy to fill your physical and energy bodies, to bring greater harmony and balance to your life. Then use the Power Symbol to bring the energy in to support the Harmony Symbol.

Let yourself stay in a meditative state and imagine being surrounded and encompassed by Reiki for at least five minutes, but preferably for about 15 minutes, or until you feel much calmer and more content. Then draw a Power Symbol to seal in the peaceful energies, saying its mantra three times. Clap your hands or shake them vigorously to break the energy connections.

For Letting Go of Blocked Feelings or Unhealthy Attachments

In a similar way to the method above, draw or imagine drawing a large Harmony Symbol over your crown chakra, then imagine the symbol expanding until it encompasses the whole of you. Say its mantra three times and ask and *intend* that it bring its gentle, healing, peaceful and restorative energy to fill your physical and energy bodies, to bring greater harmony and balance to your life.

Then use the Power Symbol, saying its mantra three times, and ask and *intend* that it work with the Harmony Symbol to unblock and release any deeply held feelings (such as resentment or hatred), or that it unblock and release any unhealthy attachments (for example, to a former husband/wife/boyfriend/girlfriend).

It is helpful if you can visualize something like a small cloud of gray energy, representing all your old emotions related to this situation, actually being detached and floating up through your energy field to be released—imagine it going "pop" as it moves outside your aura—to be healed by Reiki. When you feel calmer and more content, draw a Power Symbol to seal out the old, useless emotions, saying its mantra three times, then clap your hands or shake them vigorously to break the energy connections.

SENDING REIKI INTO THE PAST

You can send Reiki into the past, to allow it to heal past events or hurts. It will not necessarily physically alter what has happened—although it can have an impact energetically—but it can allow healing and forgiveness to permeate that time, which will gently alter the way you feel about it.

For example, if you had a difficult or traumatic experience in the past and you know the approximate date, you can use the Distant Symbol to send Reiki back to that time to heal the problem or trauma. It often helps if you have a photograph of yourself close to the time of the event in question, but if you don't know the date or don't have a photograph, it will still work by simply naming the problem and asking that Reiki go to the cause and heal it.

1. Write down the situation and roughly the timing (for example, a broken relationship when you were 20 years old) and draw or imagine the Distant Healing Symbol over the paper (and photograph of you at that age, if you have one). Silently say its sacred mantra three times, sensing it connecting the you of today with the you of that time.

2. Draw or imagine the Harmony Symbol over the paper/ photograph, and say its mantra three times, sensing its healing flowing to the hurt and upset and to the root cause and the lessons you were meant to learn from the event.

3. Draw or imagine the Power Symbol over the paper/photograph, and say its mantra three times, sensing a strong flow of Reiki moving into that time.

4. Allow the Reiki to flow for 15 to 20 minutes, or longer if it feels appropriate. Then draw the Power Symbol over the paper/ photograph, and say its mantra three times, *intending* that the healing be sealed in. Then clap your hands to break the connection, and let go of that event in your thoughts.

If in the days following this activity you get a sense that the healing is not complete—perhaps you have dreamed about the event, or it unexpectedly enters your thoughts quite a few times—then repeat the above instructions, sending Reiki again to the same situation. You can do this as many times as you feel is needed, but once is often enough. However, sometimes it is the way you have worded the situation that is preventing the healing from being completed. For example, perhaps you are trying to send the Reiki to the other person involved, which ethically is not the correct way to do this.

You can only have responsibility for your own self-healing, but by healing your own reactions and thoughts about a particular time or event, that healing automatically flows outward rather like the ripples made by a pebble thrown into a pond. It gradually permeates through the energetic signature of the whole situation, including allowing any other people involved to receive whatever healing their Higher Selves deem is necessary.

So healing your own part in the event can have some extraordinary effects—I have known cases where family members, who have not spoken to each other for years because of a family feud, have suddenly got in touch again when students of mine sent Reiki to the original situation—healing their *own* feelings about it helped others to recognize this on a subconscious, energetic level, so that they too could heal their own part in it.

SENDING REIKI INTO THE FUTURE

It is simple to send Reiki into the future. If you know you will be involved in an important event, situation or activity in the future with which you feel you need Reiki's help, such as a job interview, a visit to the dentist or a potentially difficult business meeting, write down the event or situation and the approximate date and time.

Proceed in the same way as above, sensing the Reiki flowing into the future to wait for you there. It is also possible to "bank" Reiki so that you can draw on it as and when you need it, by imagining some sort of container—it could be a box, a jug or a fun container like a big piggy bank.

1. Draw the Distant Symbol to connect to the container, saying its sacred mantra three times, then draw the Power Symbol.

2. Say its mantra three times and visualize the container filling up with Reiki, for the highest and greatest good.

When it is used in this way, the Reiki energy stores up like a battery. When the time comes, its healing energy descends to surround you and help you. People have used this technique to help them with all sorts of events, including driving tests, trips to meet their potential mother-in-law, hospital appointments— basically anything that might be difficult or frightening or that would make them feel nervous, as well as happier events like weddings, parties, the first day in a new job and so on. Just try it out for yourself.

EMPOWERING EVERYTHING IN YOUR LIFE

There is really no limit to the ways in which you can use the Reiki Symbols to enhance and empower your life. The simplest and easiest thing to do is to use the Power Symbol regularly over just about everything, with the intention of filling it with Reiki so that not only will it function even more effectively, but it will also emanate Reiki, so that as you walk around your home or other spaces you regularly use, you are always soaking up Reiki. The following is a sample list, but you can probably think of even more. Just be creative, and enjoy it:

- Bathwater
- Lightbulbs/heaters
- Boiler
- Showerhead
- Television/radio
- Oven/microwave
- Toiletries
- CD/cassette player
- Washing machine/dryer
- Cosmetics
- Computer/laptop/electronic diary
- Dishwasher/vacuum cleaner

- Clothes
- Telephone/cell phone/pager
- Teapot/coffeemaker
- Jewelry/clocks/watches
- Car/motorcycle/bicycle
- Food processor/juicer
- Bed/pillows
- Chairs/sofa/dining table
- ... and anything else!

Now you have lots of practical ways of using the symbols to enhance your life, and I hope you will find them really helpful. However, it is now time to be a bit more adventurous, so the next chapter has some very creative ways of using your Second Degree skills to have fun with Reiki. Enjoy!

Chapter 14

Creative Uses for Your Second Degree Skills

Now is the time to start having fun with Reiki. The symbols are so versatile that the only limits will be how much imagination you can bring to using Reiki.

ENHANCING INTUITION AND PSYCHIC ABILITY

Everyone has some form of psychic ability that they can choose to develop or block. However, being attuned to Reiki can often unblock this ability or allow you to develop it further than you would otherwise have done. This is not anything to be nervous about because, as always, Reiki works only for the highest and greatest good, so if it is the right time in your spiritual journey for you to develop your intuitive skills, you will be able to do so.

There are three types of psychic ability:

1. Clairsentience, meaning "clear sensing," to feel or sense subtle energies or spirit.

2. Clairaudience, meaning "clear hearing," such as in mediumship or channeling.

3. Clairvoyance, meaning "clear sight," such as being able to see into the future and the past and being able to see subtle energies like auras.

Clairsentience

Many people who do Reiki find their ability to sense subtle energies greatly improves as their experience with Reiki increases. They can detect different layers of people's auras and sense imbalances, and also check whether those imbalances have dispersed after giving Reiki. Also, they become more aware of any "atmosphere" in a room or between people. Some build up their skills so that they can sense the presence of spiritual beings, including spirit guides and angels, even to the extent of being able to feel their touch.

Clairaudience

Other people find that they become mediums: hearing messages from discarnate beings (that is, people who are no longer living on the physical plane) or develop the ability to "hear" guidance from their spirit guides (discarnate beings in a higher dimension who wish to share their wisdom to help us). They may also be able to "channel" information from highly evolved teachers from spiritual realms (sometimes called ascended masters).

Some people actually hear real voices that seem to come from outside their heads, but most just find that the words appear inside their heads, like thoughts—and yet not quite like thoughts. I know that may be confusing, but it is quite difficult to describe. One way to tell the difference is that when a question is being asked—even if you are doing the asking yourself—the answer appears in your head before you have even finished formulating the question.

Clairvoyance

Quite often, people develop the ability to "see" other realities—for instance, they are able to see inside someone's body to tell what is wrong with them physically. The first time this happens can be a big shock: I remember my first occasion, which was seeing someone's cardiovascular system in full moving Technicolor, with three blockages clearly apparent, and wow, was I surprised! However, it did mean that I could position my hands directly over the blockages and that I could check afterward to see if the blockages had gone—which they had.

Other clairvoyant abilities include seeing colors or blockages in auras and chakras; "seeing" the energy representations of a person's life within their aura—for example, what their home looks like or being able to describe their family members—and being able to see visions of things that have happened in the past or that might happen in the future. (Note that I said "might" happen in the future. Your future is not fixed, as it is being created by your own thoughts. So if you change your mind, you will change your future too.) Some people also develop the ability to see angels and spirit guides.

HOW TO DEVELOP PSYCHIC AWARENESS

If you wish to develop your psychic awareness and intuitive skills further, work with the Reiki symbols on your third eye (brow chakra), the seat of your intuition, inspiration and insight:

1. Draw both the Power Symbol and the Harmony Symbol onto each hand.

2. Hold one hand on your forehead and the other hand behind your head at approximately the same level.

3. Alternatively, draw both symbols actually on your forehead, or in your aura, about 5 cm (2 in) away from your third eye chakra.

4. *Intend* that Reiki should flow into your third eye to awaken and enhance your intuitive ability safely and easily, for your highest and greatest good.

5. Then hold your hands on your head for a few minutes, allowing the Reiki to flow.

Don't do this too often or for too long, as you may get headaches. If you don't feel comfortable doing this, write on a piece of paper "I wish to develop my psychic awareness safely and easily for my highest and greatest good." Hold the paper between your hands and place the symbols over it or put it in the center of a crystal grid (see page 214).

PSYCHIC PROTECTION

It is very important to protect yourself psychically as you become more sensitive and intuitive, because as the vibrational frequencies of your energy body are raised, they become more attractive to some of the lower energies. This can make you more vulnerable than usual to psychic drains (people who drain your energy, whether they know they are doing this or not) and psychic attack (harmful thoughts from other people, again, whether they know they are doing this or not). Here are some suggestions for self-protection, and it is a good idea to carry out at least one of them at the beginning and end of every day.

- Draw a large Power Symbol in front of you and step into it, saying its mantra three times. Imagine being wrapped inside the Power Symbol so that it is in front, behind and on each side of you, and *intend* that the Reiki protect you from any negativity or harm.

- Imagine yourself in a bubble of white or golden light that is filled with Reiki; *intend* that the edges of the bubble are permeable only by love, light, Reiki and positive energies.

- Imagine yourself inside a bubble of Reiki light, and imagine that the bubble is closely surrounded by a fine mesh made of gold which is only permeable by love, light, Reiki and positive energies.

- If you ever feel really threatened, then do all of the above. Outside your bubble of light filled with Reiki and covered with gold mesh, imagine a ring of fire. Outside that imagine a shiny eggshell made of mirror or shiny silver, with the mirrored side facing outward. This effectively forms an energetic boundary around you, so that any negativity or psychic attack sent your way will only rebound to the sender, because it is reflected by the mirror or silver.

EARTH HEALING AND USING REIKI
ON WORLD SITUATIONS AND DISASTERS

The Earth really needs as much healing as we can give her, and with Reiki you have a wonderful tool to use both for planetary healing and for sending healing to world situations or to help in crises or disasters. There are many methods for Earth healing, and some suggestions follow that can all be enhanced by using Reiki.

- Go to a place of power, such as an ancient stone circle, and visualize a huge Power Symbol over the top of the circle. Either sit in the middle or place your hands on one of the stones, and allow Reiki to flow into the stone and then around the circle and into the earth itself.

- Another good thing to do at a stone circle or ancient cairn is to "walk" the shape of the Power Symbol into the earth—although of course you really need to be alone to do this, as the symbol's shape is meant to be kept secret.

- Sit or stand either outdoors or indoors and draw or imagine a large Power Symbol over the earth or floor. Then, with your palms facing downward, direct Reiki into the earth.

- Imagine that you are holding a small version of the world between your hands, and send it Reiki. (Use the Distant Symbol to connect you to the Earth, and then the Power Symbol to activate greater healing.)

- Hold something in your hands to represent the Earth, such as a stone, and draw the Power Symbol over it, filling it with Reiki, and *intending* that the Reiki should fill the planet.

- To send Reiki to global situations, such as famines, ecological disasters or war zones, write down the situation and hold the piece of paper in your hands. Draw the Distant Symbol, then the Harmony Symbol and then the Power Symbol, saying each of their sacred mantras three times and *intending* that Reiki should go to that situation for the highest possible good. In this way the Reiki is not being constrained to go to only one aspect of the situation, such as the people affected by the famine, but to the whole, so that it can also permeate the aid agencies, the governments, any warring factions, and so on.

It really is gratifying to feel that you can do *something* to help, because so often we are too far removed from such situations to either fully understand them or to offer practical assistance. However, by sending Reiki we cannot predetermine the outcome, but must trust Reiki to work with the Higher Consciousness to heal, harmonize and balance the situation for the highest and greatest good.

USING REIKI WITH CRYSTALS

Crystals and gems have been regarded in many cultures as having magical powers and have been used throughout history for their healing qualities and beauty. Each crystal has different energy balancing and vibrational qualities. These can interact with the human energy body to promote healing, which is enhanced even more by filling them with Reiki. Using Reiki with crystals is not a part of traditional Reiki, but many Masters and Practitioners find crystals a useful and attractive addition to their healing work.

Types of Crystal

Most of the popular crystals are forms of quartz, and their unique crystalline structure seems to be ideally suited to holding healing energy. There are many different types and shapes of crystal, and most can be used as a vibrational tool to dislodge negative vibrations, the most commonly used for this purpose being clear quartz, rose quartz and amethyst. When choosing your crystals, hold the intent or purpose of "healing" in your mind as you select them.

Clear Quartz

This is the most versatile and most easily programmable crystal. It receives, activates, contains, amplifies and transmits energy, balancing the chakras and dispelling negativity from your own energy field and from the environment. When used as a tool for therapy it is an excellent channeler of healing energy. It is also known to promote clear-sightedness and inspire communication with your Higher Self, and it works well with any area of the body.

Rose Quartz

This is known as the "love stone," because its energies promote forgiveness and compassion by helping you to let go of stored anger, resentment, guilt, fear and jealousy. It eases emotional and sexual imbalance and enhances awareness of your true self, helping you to learn to love yourself. It works particularly well with the spleen, kidneys, heart, circulatory system and reproductive system.

Amethyst

This is known as "the elevator" because it is a powerful aid to spiritual enhancement, cutting through illusion and inspiring healing, divine love, inspiration and intuition. It also strengthens the endocrine and immune systems and has a good effect on right-brain activity (the creative and intuitive side) and the pineal and pituitary glands, and is believed to be an exceptional blood cleanser and energizer.

Some crystals can be found in their original rough state, while others have been shaped or polished. For healing I don't think it matters what shape you use, but I do find crystal pyramids, crystal balls and crystal wands particularly useful, as they seem to concentrate healing energy most effectively.

Cleansing

When you first bring the crystals home it is important to cleanse them thoroughly. This is because they absorb energy easily, and you don't know what kinds of energy they have been absorbing before you bought them. Cleansing rids them of any negative energetic vibrations.

There are various methods of cleansing, such as holding the crystals in running water (not salt water) and letting them dry naturally afterward, and by leaving them in bright sunlight or moonlight so that they absorb a full charge of masculine (Sun) and feminine (Moon) energies. I use this method, but I also use Reiki. Simply hold the crystal in your hands and/or draw the Power Symbol over it, say the mantra three times and *intend* that Reiki should cleanse the crystal.

To empower and program your crystals once they have been thoroughly cleansed, pick up all the crystals individually and draw all three Reiki symbols over them, saying their sacred mantras and *intending* that the crystals be filled with an unlimited supply of Reiki. This will then be held within the crystals and released when required to be used for healing.

You can carry a crystal around with you to aid your own healing or give it to someone else who needs healing energy. I don't use crystals during a Reiki treatment, but some people like to place charged crystals (that is, ones filled with Reiki) near a client, or even on the client's chakras, during a treatment. If this is something you would like to try, I would recommend you attend a course on crystal healing to find out more about them, and of course it would be important to ascertain if the client was happy with using them. You should remove the crystals before smoothing the aura down.

You can also write down any problem you are experiencing on a piece of paper and place it under a programed crystal, intending that the Reiki flow constantly into the problem to promote healing for the highest and greatest good. It is best to cleanse the crystal and reprogram it once a week to maintain the strength of the energy.

Creating a Crystal Grid

Placing charged crystals in a grid formation magnifies their power in a similar way to many people treating one person with Reiki: the energy increases exponentially. There are a number of ways in which you can create crystal grids, but all have a central crystal and a number of crystals surrounding it.

Clear quartz crystals normally have one end where the facets end in a point, so these are the ones I usually use. Placing the points facing toward the center concentrates the energy in the center of the grid, while placing the points facing outward allows the energy to dissipate over a wide area. Sometimes it is possible to obtain crystals with points at both ends so they would transmit energy in both directions.

Crystal grids create a powerful space for healing. They can be any size you want, but the most useful size is up to a diameter of 30 cm (12 in) for indoor use. You can create a small crystal grid almost anywhere, but it is best to keep it out of sight or out of reach of other people once it has been set up, because its energy will dissipate if it is disturbed.

The crystals can be placed on a cloth, a board or a tray if you want them to be portable, or on a high window ledge or shelf if they can stay in the same place for a long time. To permeate or protect a sizeable area with Reiki you can create a large grid by placing crystals in the corners of a room or in each corner of your home, or buried in the ground at each corner of your garden, for example. However, just because the grid is large it does not mean the crystals have to be. For most purposes, crystals about 5 to 10 cm (2 to 4 in) in length are fine.

Before setting up the grid I would always cleanse the area first, physically and energetically, and it is important to do this regularly.

To allow the grid to become dusty would be disrespectful of the healing properties of both the crystals and the Reiki.

Once a crystal grid has been set up it can be left where it is for a long time, providing you remember to clean and cleanse the area and the crystals regularly and re-empower the grid with Reiki when you put the crystals back in place. My Reiki Master, William Rand, has placed 12-point crystal grids fixed on copper plates at the North and South Poles, designated for Earth healing and world peace. They will presumably stay there for as long as the copper and crystals continue to exist. Even though they may now be under many feet of snow or ice, they can still be regularly recharged with Reiki using the Distant Symbol to connect with each of them.

The main way to use a crystal grid is to place under the central crystal something that represents what you want the healing to go to—for example, a photograph or a piece of paper with a name on it. It will then receive continuous Reiki, although you will need to "top up" the Reiki regularly and will also need to gently cleanse all the crystals regularly. You can therefore use the grids to empower affirmations; to send distant healing to an individual or to a list of people; to send healing to a single situation or multiple situations; to send Reiki to a future or past event; and so on.

Four-point Crystal Grid

This simple grid is especially good for Earth healing, as the four crystals can represent north, south, east and west, and the central crystal can represent the whole Earth—a crystal sphere would be particularly appropriate here. However, it can also be used for other healing purposes: placed around your home or your therapy room to create a healing environment, or as a small grid to use for distant healing of people, places or situations.

Cleanse and empower each crystal as above, placing a crystal in the center (any shape will do, but apart from a sphere a pyramid is particularly good, as its base has four sides) and place the other four crystals with their pointed ends facing the center.

Draw the Power Symbol over the grid, making sure you encompass the whole grid, say its mantra three times and *intend* to empower this grid with unlimited Reiki energy (you can add the other two symbols as well, if you wish). *Intend* that whatever is represented by what is placed in the center should receive healing (for example, a photograph or a piece of paper with a name on it is a representation of the person, not the actual person).

Eight-point Crystal Grid

This grid can be any size you choose and is also very good for Earth healing or for world situations, as it has a crystal in each of the eight directions (that is, including SE, SW, NE and NW), but it can be used for more general healing too. Cleanse all your crystals, then place a crystal in the center and eight evenly spaced crystals around it with the points facing inward toward the central crystal.

Intend to create a healing crystal grid, and empower the grid first with the Distant Symbol to enable the grid to connect even more effectively with whatever is placed within it; then the Harmony Symbol, to generate deep healing and harmony; then the Power Symbol to bring in the Reiki, saying their sacred mantras three times each. Top up the grid with the Power Symbol every day if possible, and cleanse all the crystals thoroughly at least once every three weeks. (The grid can then be set up again.)

Twelve-point Crystal Grid

This is especially good for distant healing where you want the healing to continue to go to someone (or several people) for a number of days or even weeks. Place a crystal in the center and then 12 equally spaced crystals in a circle around it, like the numbers on a clock face. Empower the grid with the three Reiki symbols, as in the eight-point grid above.

When placing a photograph or name of a person in the grid, as you draw the Distant Symbol say its mantra three times, then the name of the person three times, their location once and the number of days/nights the healing is to flow. Then draw the Power Symbol over it, saying its mantra three times. Always remember to add "for the greatest and highest good" for all distant healing.

As you can see, there is a lot of scope for using your Second Degree skills in all sorts of creative ways. In Part IV, however, you will be introduced to the newly rediscovered techniques from the Japanese tradition, which will add another interesting dimension to your healing abilities.

Part IV

The Japanese Tradition

Chapter 15

The Importance of Self-Cleansing

As you progress on your spiritual path with Reiki, you become increasingly sensitive to other people's energies, and one of the possible consequences of this is that you can "pick up" energy—particularly negative energy—from other people and from your surroundings. Of course you can protect yourself from this, as I have discussed previously, but I am sure you don't want to be a kind of psychic blotting paper, walking around absorbing everybody else's rubbish! It is therefore *vital* to cleanse yourself (your whole energy body as well as your physical body) every day, and often several times a day, depending upon what you are doing.

My initial impression when I was trained was that the Reiki channel created by an attunement could not become blocked, but after many years of experience I have revised my opinion on this. I now realize that unless people work on themselves by using a regular energy-cleansing routine and carrying out a self-treatment each day, plus working on their spiritual awareness and development, the Reiki channel does seem to get smaller, which affects the amount of flow. Energy meridians are in this way not dissimilar to a water pipe that can become clogged by a buildup of residues on the inside of the pipe, slowing down the flow. If the residues continue to accumulate and nothing is done to clean the pipe out, it could eventually become completely blocked.

I am convinced that this is one of the main reasons why, in Japan, students receive regular *Rei-ju* empowerments, not only to increase the amount of Reiki they can channel, but also to help to keep their energy channels free-flowing. Reiki itself will cut through negative energy and other blockages, but it needs as clear a channel as possible to work effectively, and most of us have plenty of negative "stuff" stored in our bodies. Some of this could possibly adhere to the Reiki channel as it is loosened and brought to the surface to be eliminated over the weeks, months and years of using Reiki. Negativity in the form of thoughts and emotions is pretty stubborn stuff!

Eventually our energy channels can become really clean and free-flowing, but how long this takes will depend upon how much "baggage" we have been collecting during our lifetime(s). However, the process is ongoing and continuous. Having Reiki does not shield us forever from susceptibility to collecting negative thoughts and emotions. Our initial attunement starts the purification process, but afterward we really need to continue with self-treatments, a sensible energy-cleansing routine and, if possible, regular *Rei-ju* empowerments.

One of the main aspects that has been missing in the Reiki traditions in the West has been self-cleansing, and of course it is clear to us now that Dr. Usui would have been well aware of the need for energetic cleansing because of his knowledge of martial arts with the consequent emphasis on keeping the *Ki* healthy and free-flowing. With hindsight it is probably not surprising that he included in his healing system a number of techniques that are similar to those from the *chi kung* (*Ki-Ko*) traditions for energy raising and balancing.

GASSHO

First an explanation of *Gassho*, which you will have seen mentioned briefly before in this book: the word itself literally means "to place the two palms together," and it is probably the most fundamental of all the *mudras* (symbolic hand gestures or positions) that we use. It is a gesture of respect, humility and reverence, and is used to concentrate the mind and to express the total unity of Being. It is seen as a connection between body, mind and spirit, promoting calmness. In Reiki it is used during the Japanese empowerment called *Rei-ju* and during the Western tradition attunement process. It can be used to begin and end any of the techniques in this book, as a sign of prayerful respect and honor of the system, the energy, the client and all creation.

To make a *Gassho*, place both hands together with their palms touching and the fingers and thumbs close together and extended upward in a prayer position, and hold them so that the thumbs are held close to the center of the chest (heart chakra). After a few moments, keeping your hands together, bow slightly to show respect.

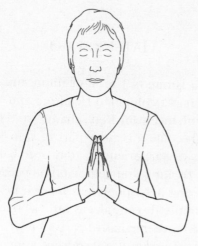

Gassho *hand position.*

JAPANESE TECHNIQUES FOR SELF-CLEANSING

The first three techniques for self-cleansing come from the Japanese tradition. The *Hatsurei-ho*, which is a combination of energy cleansing and meditation techniques, can become a vital part of your everyday cleansing armory. I now recommend to my students that they do this at the start of every day and then again before going to bed at night. Part of the *Hatsurei-ho*, called *Kenyoku-ho* (Dry Brushing), can be used on its own as a way of brushing off negative energies. Another technique, called the Reiki Shower, floods your energy field with Reiki to cleanse and revitalize it. Both of these methods can be used as and when they are needed.

If you are treating clients, I would suggest you carry out a full *Hatsurei-ho* before the first client and after the last client, and do the

Dry Brushing technique or the Reiki Shower technique between each two. After the last client, a cold shower—quickly followed by a nice warm one if you wish—is the best way to rid yourself of any residual negativity and prepare you for the rest of your day or evening.

None of these techniques requires you to use the Reiki Symbols, so anyone with any level of Reiki can use them. However, if you have Second Degree you can draw a Power Symbol over each hand before you start, intending that Reiki should flow to clear and cleanse your energy body, which can enhance the process.

HATSUREI-HO

I think *Hatsurei-ho* is one of the most important of the Japanese Reiki techniques. It is a combined cleansing and meditation practice that helps to enhance your Reiki channel and help you to grow spiritually. It can become a regular part of your spiritual practice and is an ideal way to start or end the day or to begin your practice of Reiki, whether treating yourself or other people. Although the length of the following description may make it look complicated, it is actually quite simple. It can take as little as ten minutes, or you can stretch out the more meditative parts of it (*Joshin Kokyu Ho*: the cleansing breath, and *Seishin Toitsu*: concentration or meditation) to half an hour or more—it is up to you.

Kihon Shisei—Standard Posture

First make yourself comfortable in a sitting position either on the floor or on a chair, then allow yourself to relax and close your eyes. Focus your attention on your *Tan-dien*, an energy point that is between 3 and 5 cm (1 and 2 in) below your navel. With your hands on your lap, palms facing downward, spend a few moments concentrating on bringing your breath into a slow, steady rhythm as you center yourself and focus your thoughts, and *intend* to begin the *Hatsurei-ho*.

Kenyoku-ho—Dry Bathing or Brushing

The brushing can be done either with contact, touching the body, or more easily without contact about 5 cm (2 in) away from your body, in the aura. Each of the movements is completed quite quickly. Focus on your breath for this exercise, breathing out as you brush and making a sound as you exhale, such as "haaah."

1. Place the fingers of your right hand at the point where your collarbone meets your left shoulder, with your hand lying flat, fingers and thumb close together.

2. Draw the flat hand down with a quick, sweeping movement diagonally across your chest in a straight line, from your left shoulder down to your right hip. At the same time, expel your breath quickly, making a definite sound throughout the movement, for example "haaah."

3. Now do the same thing on the other side, placing your left hand on your right shoulder, fingertips by the collarbone, and brush down from the right shoulder to the left hip, again exhaling loudly.

4. Return your right hand to your left shoulder and repeat the process again, with your right hand brushing diagonally from your left shoulder to your right hip while exhaling loudly.

5. Next you are going to repeat the process, but this time instead of brushing diagonally across your body, you will be brushing along your arms from shoulder to fingertips. Place your right hand on the edge of your left shoulder, with your hand flat and your fingertips just on the edge of the shoulder, pointing slightly outward.

6. Keeping your left arm straight and at your side, sweep your right hand quickly down the outside of your left arm, all the way to the fingertips of your left hand. At the same time, expel your breath quickly and loudly as before, making a definite sound throughout the movement.

7. Repeat this process on the other side, with your left hand on your right shoulder, brushing down quickly to the fingertips of your right hand, and expelling your breath loudly as before.

8. Complete this process by once more sweeping your right hand down your left arm from shoulder to fingertips, again exhaling loudly.

Connect to Reiki

Now raise both your hands in the air above your head with your palms facing each other about 20 to 30 cm (8 to 12 in) apart, and visualize and feel the light and vibration of Reiki flowing into and between your hands and running through your whole body. When you can sense this vibration, continue with the next section.

Joshin Kokyu Ho—Cleansing Breath

1. Now lower your arms and put your hands on your lap with your palms facing upward, and breathe naturally and steadily through your nose. Begin to focus your attention on your Hara line (a major energy line running through the center of your body, connecting all the major chakras from the root to the crown) and allow your body to relax.

2. Concentrate on your breathing, and as you breathe in visualize Reiki as white light pouring in through your crown chakra into your Reiki channel and down the Hara line through your major chakras. Then imagine the Reiki spreading out, expanding to fill the whole of your body from your head to your toes and from your shoulders to your fingertips, and sense it melting all your tensions away.

3. As you breathe out visualize the Reiki light, which is filling your whole body, beginning to expand so that it flows through your skin, spreading out to fill your aura, and then imagine it flowing beyond your aura in all directions to infinity.

4. Continue this process for a few minutes, or as long as you wish, breathing Reiki in and out.

Gassho

When you feel ready put your hands together in the *Gassho* (prayer) position in front of the center of your chest, at about the level of your heart chakra.

Seishin Toitsu—Concentration or Meditation

1. Keeping your hands in the *Gassho* position, take your focus away from breathing through your nose and imagine that you are breathing through your hands.

2. As you breathe in, visualize the light of Reiki flowing in through your hands, and from there into your heart chakra. Imagine it filling your heart chakra and then sense it flowing into your Hara line. Visualize it flowing up and down your Hara line until it is filled with white light.

3. Then, as you breathe out, visualize that the light, which now fills your Hara line, is radiating out again through your hands, flowing out and spreading Reiki in all directions around the world and into the Universe.

4. Continue this process for a few minutes or as long as you wish, breathing in Reiki through your hands, into your Hara line and out of your hands again, then let your mind settle into a peaceful, meditative state. (If you are undertaking this practice with other Reiki students and your Reiki Master, this is the time when you would normally receive the *Rei-ju* empowerment, so you would remain still with your eyes closed until your Reiki Master informed you that the *Rei-ju* was completed.)

Gokai Sansho

In the traditional way, Japanese Reiki students would at this point say the Reiki Principles aloud three times. You may feel that you would like to do the same, so you can either use the translation on page 13 or one of the versions based on what Mrs. Takata taught on page 253 and suit.

Mokunen

1. Place your hands back onto your lap with palms facing downward, and *intend* that the *Hatsurei-ho* be completed.

2. When you feel ready, open your eyes and shake your hands gently up and down and then from left to right for a few seconds, to bring you back to a greater state of physical awareness.

You are now ready to get on with your day, or to begin your practice of Reiki either as a self-treatment or for the treatment of others.

KENYOKU-HO—DRY BATHING OR BRUSHING OFF

This is part of the *Hatsurei-ho* (see page 222), but it can be done separately either on its own or before the Reiki Shower technique below. This brushing off is useful to do as you step into your shower before you turn on the water, because then the water will wash away all the negative energy that has been brushed off; but don't do it when you step into a bath or all the "gunk" you have just brushed off will go into the water, which you will then be splashing all over yourself again.

One thing you will notice is that there is an uneven number of actions in each part—brushing the energy twice as often from the left shoulder downward, as from the right shoulder. My normal reaction would be to "even out" the strokes, so that both sides would be treated the same, but apparently the Japanese are superstitious about the number 4, as the word is the same as the word for "death," so they prefer not to do things four times!

THE REIKI SHOWER TECHNIQUE

This is a technique from the Japanese tradition that is suitable for anyone with any level of Reiki. It consists of activating and cleansing your whole energy body by absorbing Reiki energy throughout the body like a shower. You can use this technique almost anywhere for cleansing yourself. It also helps to center yourself, raising your consciousness and bringing you into a meditative state.

1. Stand or sit and make yourself comfortable. Close or half-close your eyes and begin to slow down and deepen your breathing until you can maintain a naturally slow and steady pace.

2. Place your hands in the *Gassho* position. Stay like this for a few moments, and *intend* to use Reiki to cleanse and activate your energy body.

3. Then separate your hands and lift them above your head, as high as possible, keeping them about 20 to 30 cm (8 to 12 in)

apart. Wait for a few moments until you begin to feel the Reiki building up between your hands, then turn your palms downward so that they are facing the top of your head.

4. Visualize and *intend* that you are receiving a shower of Reiki energy from the palms of your hands that flows over and through your whole physical and energy body, cleansing you and removing any negative energy. If you have Second Degree Reiki, you can imagine an image of the Power Symbol flowing through you if you wish. Say its mantra three times, imagining it vibrating throughout your energy body. Similarly, if you have Third Degree Reiki you can use the Master Symbol and its mantra in the same way.

5. When you feel the vibration of the Reiki energy flowing over and through you, move your hands, palms still facing toward you, and begin to draw them slowly down over your face and in front of your body, keeping your hands about 20 to 30 cm (8 to 12 in) away from the body. *Intend* that Reiki is flowing from your hands and continuing to cleanse and revitalize you as you draw your hands all the way down your body and then down your legs to your feet. Eventually turn your palms to face the floor and gently throw the energy off your hands so that any negative energy flows out of your feet and into the earth below, where it can be transformed and used by the planet.

6. Repeat this exercise a few times—I find three times to be ideal—and you should feel cleansed, revitalized and more alive as Reiki healing and light flows into all of your cells and fills every part of your body.

7. Place your hands together again in the *Gassho* position and spend a few moments experiencing gratitude for the Reiki, then finish. You may find it helpful to clap your hands once or twice to help you to return to a more wakeful state if this exercise leaves you feeling a bit "spaced."

8. After completing the Reiki Shower your whole body is activated with Reiki, your hands are filled with the light of Reiki and you are ready to carry out healing for yourself and/or for others.

Using Cold Showers for Self-Cleansing

To cleanse your physical and energy bodies fully, I recommend a cold shower. Yes, I know it might be an unpleasant thought, but it really works! However, if you have any health condition that might make you particularly susceptible to shock from the cold water please ask your doctor before adding this technique to your cleansing routine.

Cold water has a particularly vibrant cleansing energy, so when it flows through your energy field and over your physical body the "shock" of it shakes loose the negative or "sticky" energy that is trapped in and around your body. While a warm or hot shower or bath is good for cleaning your physical body and can also be very relaxing, it has the effect of expanding your aura. This can potentially make the negative, sticky energy enter farther into your energy body so that it becomes harder to remove. This therefore means that it is important to *start* your shower with cold water rather than ending with it, which some people like to do to close the pores in the skin, although you can do *both* if you wish.

The important thing is to let the cold water flow over all your chakras, so that they are cleansed. You don't necessarily have to stand right under the showerhead with the cold water flowing over all of you at once, unless you want to, and you can wear a shower cap unless you want to wash your hair. Your crown chakra will still be cleansed by the water flowing over the cap. Also, it is only necessary to be under the cold water for about ten seconds in total.

The parts that need the water to flow over them are all your major chakras at the front from the crown down to the root chakra and the same down the back, plus the minor chakras and major points on your meridian system, including your shoulders, elbows, wrists, hands, hips, knees, ankles and feet. You might find it easiest to hold the showerhead in your hand and direct the water quickly, always in a downward flow—I usually start with my feet, just to get used to the temperature, then move to each shoulder, down each arm and then down each side of the body. Then I let the water flow from the crown of my head down the center of my back, and then from the crown down the front of my face, throat and body, finishing with both legs and feet again. As soon as this is accomplished you can turn the water up to the nice, warm temperature you usually shower with, and I guarantee that you will feel wonderfully clean, invigorated and refreshed.

If you don't have a shower in your home, you can buy shower attachments that will fit onto most bath taps, or you can use a pitcher: just fill the pitcher with cold water, stand in the bath, and pour the water over your chakras. Afterward, you can fill the pitcher with comfortably hot water, to warm yourself up, although a vigorous toweling or wrapping yourself in a toweling robe will do the job too.

I recommend at least two cold showers a day—one in the morning, to wash off any negative energy you have picked up during the night (at least a part of our spirit rises out of our body during our sleep, but even if this does not happen, any negative thoughts or dreams can "pollute" our energy field), then another one before bed, to wash off the negative "stuff" we pick up during an average day. This includes the energetic residue of any arguments or disagreements, negative comments and thoughts from people we have met, or even the misery and violence we have seen on a television news program.

If you work in any of the caring professions, or as a therapist or counselor, or in any profession where you are dealing with negative people, I really recommend a cold shower as soon as you get in from work; otherwise the negative energy you have been absorbing all day from your clients will slowly seep into that nice, comfortable chair into which you flop as soon as you get home. Much better to wash it all off, put on clean clothes and feel refreshed and ready to enjoy your evening.

If after reading this you suddenly think of all the negative energy that you must have brought into your home over the years—don't panic! Use the Power Symbol all over the home—chairs, sofas, beds, as well as the corners, walls, floors and ceilings of all the rooms—with the intention of cleansing all negative energy.

If you have not done Reiki 2, just sit quietly with your palms open on your lap. Allow and *intend* that Reiki should flow around your home to cleanse the energies, and visualize the Reiki spreading like a white light until your home is filled with it. Over a period of weeks you will gradually sense a lighter feel as the Reiki peels away layers of negativity that have just been lying around for ages.

USING REIKI WITH YOUR NORMAL
CLEANSING ROUTINE

In addition to the above cold showers, I am sure you will continue with your usual cleansing routine—nice, relaxing hot baths and exhilarating hot showers are two of life's great pleasures, I think. However, to cleanse yourself energetically as well, you can draw the Power Symbol over the showerhead, so that as the water flows through it, it picks up Reiki to cleanse and heal you as you shower.

You can also draw the Power Symbol over your bathwater, before you step in (or when you are sitting in it, if you forget) so that you are bathing in cleansing, healing water. Add a few drops of lavender oil, light some candles, and you have the perfect remedial, relaxing retreat. (Remember, you should never leave a burning candle unattended.)

The self-cleansing techniques in this chapter are excellent ways of keeping your energy body clear so that Reiki can flow through you more effectively, and ideally you can integrate them into your daily Reiki practice. In the next chapter we discover some exciting "new" methods from the Reiki traditions in Japan, which can give your Reiki practice an added dimension.

Chapter 16

Additional Techniques from the Japanese Tradition

Because of the research that has been done in Japan (see chapter 1) we now know that Dr. Usui left a rich heritage of healing techniques that have been passed down from his *Shinpi-den* students in Japan (a *Shinpi-den* is the equivalent of a Western Reiki Master). It is believed that most of the following techniques were part of Dr. Usui's original system, the Usui Reiki Ryoho, or Usui Teate, meaning "hand touch" or "hand healing," and some of them use one hand only, which seems to have been quite usual for Dr. Usui, according to his manual, the *Usui Reiki Hikkei*.

USING THE ORIGINAL USUI REIKI TECHNIQUES

These techniques don't need the Reiki symbols, although they are optional in some cases. Indeed, the symbols and their mantras were taught in Usui's original system only to open certain abilities in the students, and when those abilities were fully manifested the use of the symbols decreased until they were rarely used. In effect, the students would have "become" the energy represented by the symbols.

One thing I need to point out is that you don't have to learn the Japanese names for all these techniques unless you particularly want to. What would be much more relevant would be to integrate some or all of these methods into your general practice of Reiki. They don't have to be treated as something separate. They are certainly very useful, but not more so than any of the techniques from the Western tradition. They are just another aspect of the Usui Reiki Ryoho, Dr. Usui's simple yet powerful system of hands-on healing.

Some of the techniques are quite similar to Western techniques, such as the method of scanning the aura for energetic disturbances, while others are quite different, for example, using gentle pressure with the fingertips instead of having the hand flat against the body. So please do try them out as a part of your diverse range of techniques, perhaps adding one or two at the beginning or the end of a Reiki treatment, maybe practicing them with friends or other Reiki practitioners first. They are certainly a very valuable addition to your list of options.

A TECHNIQUE FOR DEVELOPING SENSITIVITY

This first technique encourages sensitivity in the hands, so that you can develop the ability to feel subtle energies. It is somewhat longer than the Western method, but it certainly works well, so do try it as an alternative.

1. Begin to rub your palms together until they feel hot, then the backs of your hands, then each thumb and each finger, and finally rub your palms together again.

2. Move your hands apart and shake your wrists up and down and from left to right ten times. Hold your hands with the palms facing each other about 20 cm (8 in) apart and feel the tingling sensations of the energy between your hands.

3. Bring your attention to your breath, and each time you breathe out expel the air with a "haaah" sound. Look at the space between your hands, and as you continue this deep breathing (called *Hado*) for a while, imagine that you are breathing in and out through your hands.

4. Finally, clench your hands tightly into fists and then release them.

5. Repeat steps 1 through 4 if you feel you need to, then move on to step 6.

6. Hold your hands at chest height about 20 cm (8 in) apart, and visualize or imagine that you are holding an empty balloon. With your eyes half closed, keep looking at the space between your hands, imagining the balloon there. Continue with the *Hado* breathing, breathing out with a "haaah" sound, and as you do so, feel and *intend* that the energy from your palms is going into the balloon. As you breathe Reiki into this imaginary balloon your hands move wider apart as it fills with energy and gets larger, and as you breathe in again the balloon shrinks and your hands come closer together.

7. Continue this visualization for a while and gradually the sensation of moving energy into and out of the space between your hands will become more and more real. When this happens you can change back to natural breathing. Experiment with the energy between your hands, moving your hands together, then apart, always with the palms facing each other, to sense the tingling and warmth of the energy.

8. Finally, clench your hands tightly into fists and then release them.

9. Repeat steps 6 through 8 if you feel you need to, then move on to step 10.

10. Bring your hands down toward your abdomen, and place both hands with their palms facing toward the *Tan-dien* (about 3 cm/1½ in below your navel), keeping them about 10 cm (4 in) away from your body. Feel the energy flowing from your hands into your *Tan-dien*, and keep them there until you can feel the energy quite strongly, which will mean you have built up enough sensitivity to be able to sense energy differences in different parts of your body.

11. Now slowly move your hands to other parts of your body, giving yourself time to sense the energy. Keep your palms facing your body as you slowly scan over each major chakra, from the root chakra to the crown chakra. (If you find your sensitivity becoming weaker, go back to steps 1 through 3 until the energy returns.)

12. Practice all of this activity (steps 1 through 11) from time to time until you are fully confident that you can sense energy easily and clearly.

BYOSEN REIKAN-HO

The name *Byosen Reikan-ho* means:

Byo: disease, sickness, imbalance.
Sen: before, ahead, previous, future, precedence.
Rei: energy, soul, spirit.
Kan: emotion, feeling, sensation.
Ho: treatment, method, way.

This method is similar to the "scanning" technique, and it is a way of sensing energetic imbalances with your hands, either in yourself or other people. The way in which you will sense these imbalances will vary from person to person, because it will depend on what any underlying condition is (physical or energetic), and how serious it is (and how practiced you are!). Sensations can include warmth, coolness, pulsating, piercing, stinging, throbbing, quick stabbing pain, little electric shocks, tingling or tickling, and in Japanese these feelings are called "*Hibiki.*" They normally occur only in the hands, but can occasionally be felt in the arms or even up to the shoulders in extreme cases.

Imbalances in the energy field are called "*Byosen,*" and because these occur in the aura before any physical condition presents itself, the client may not be aware of anything being wrong. Therefore if you use Reiki on those places where you sense *Byosen*, and work on it until the sensations disappear, then any potential or actual symptom or disease should be healed, or not manifest on the physical level at all. Do remember, however, that the position on the body where you feel the *Byosen* may not directly relate to the cause, as it may be linked through the energy system. For example, liver problems can sometimes cause sensations over the eyes or brow chakra.

1. Position yourself sitting or standing next to the recipient.

2. Spend a few moments centering yourself with your hands in the *Gassho* position, and allow your mind to become calm. Then *intend* to activate your intuitive ability to detect *Byosen* by saying silently to yourself "I begin *Byosen Reikan-ho* now."

3. Place your hands, palms downward, on or slightly above the recipient's body (5 to 15 cm [2 to 6 in]), starting at either the head or the feet, and begin to move them slowly down (or up) the body. Sometimes it is helpful initially to close your eyes, so that you can "tune in" more easily to any sensations in your hands. You will probably find that there is a general "background" sensation of gentle warmth or tingling or even a cool breeze when you pass your hands over one of the major chakras. However, some areas will feel different, and these are the areas of *Byosen*. The more you practice, the easier it will become to identify the subtle differences, but pay attention to changes in heat or tingling, or any of the other sensations detailed above.

4. When you sense a *Hibiki* (the sensation of *Byosen*), hold your hands on or over that area. The sensations will ebb and flow in natural cycles, increasing and then decreasing. Do not automatically assume that when the sensation reduces it is time to move your hands, as these cycles will continue for as long as your hands are on the body. The longer you hold your hands over a particular place the more energy cycles you will feel, but with each cycle the intensity diminishes. Keep your hands over the *Hibiki* for at least one cycle, and if you have time, keep your hands in the same place until there is virtually no discernible difference in sensation (that is, until there is more of a continuous sensation than an ebb and flow).

5. When you are ready, move your hands gently and slowly to the next area of *Byosen* and repeat step 4.

6. When you have completed *Byosen Reikan-ho* on the entire body remove your hands from the recipient and place them at mid-chest height in the *Gassho* position. Mentally give thanks for the Reiki, bowing slightly as a mark of respect.

REI-JI (REIJI) OR REIJI-HO

The word *Reiji-ho* means:

Rei: energy, spirit, soul
Ji: show, indicate, point out, express, display
Ho: treatment, method, way

This technique encourages relaxation, enhances your intuition and allows Reiki to guide your hands to places on the body that are in need of treatment. (In Japan they don't use the pattern of 12 or more hand positions taught in the West, as students are encouraged to develop their sensitivity and intuition by using this and the previous two techniques, so that they can place their hands wherever they intuitively sense is most in need of Reiki.) Practicing this technique will help you to expand and enhance your awareness of subtle energies.

1. Position yourself sitting or standing next to the recipient.

2. Spend a few moments centering yourself (hands in *Gassho*) and focus your attention on your *Tan-dien*, allowing your breathing to become deep and even, then *intend* to activate your intuitive ability and say silently to yourself "I begin *Reiji* now."

3. Sit or stand comfortably with your hands either palms upward on your lap or loosely by your side. Allow your body to relax completely, releasing any tensions and anxieties, and gently encourage your client to do the same. Silently call upon Reiki to fill you and your client with healing energy. Imagine Reiki flowing into you through your crown chakra, filling your whole body with healing energy, and sense it flowing out of your hands into your client's energy field, healing all levels of your being for both of you. When you feel filled with Reiki and ready to start, move on to the next step.

4. Keeping your hands in the *Gassho* position, move them up to your brow (third eye) chakra, and silently ask Reiki to direct your hands to any places on the recipient's body that need its healing energy. Wait until you feel an urge to move your hands,

as if they are being drawn by a magnet, trusting Reiki to guide them to the right places. Place your hands in whatever position they have been drawn to, with your palms either on the body or slightly above (2 to 5 cm [1 to 2 in]), and let the Reiki flow until that area has been rebalanced. When you sense that the Reiki has stopped, you will be guided to the next appropriate place, until all the parts of the body that were in need of Reiki have been balanced. The more you practice this technique, the more you will find that Reiki automatically tells you what to treat and for how long, and this intuition can be received either kinesthetically (in feelings or sensations) or mentally (thoughts, images, insights or intuitions).

5. When the Reiki stops flowing, and you are no longer being guided to any parts of your client's body, you will find that your hands will naturally return to their normal position, either beside your body, or on your knees if you are seated.

6. *Gassho*—give thanks for the Reiki and end with a bow of respect.

REIKI MAWASHI

The name *Reiki Mawashi* means:

Reiki: spiritual energy
Mawashi: round, game, revolve, current

This Reiki circle method can help to sensitize a gathering of Reiki Practitioners to feel energy flow. All the Reiki Practitioners form a circle, either sitting or standing.

1. Everyone joins hands, each person starting with their left hand under (to receive) and their right hand over (to send).

2. Keeping your hands in the same under or over position, gently loosen hands but continue to hold them 2 to 5 cm (1 to 2 in) apart from your partners on each side, so that the circle is still complete energetically but no one is touching anyone else.

3. Someone in the circle will begin the process by intending aloud that Reiki should flow, then each person begins to send Reiki flowing down their right arm and into the upturned left hand of the person on their right, so that it flows counterclockwise around the circle. As each person joins in, the Reiki moves from one hand to another, resulting in a strong current of energy around the circle that should continue for several minutes or longer if you wish.

4. When the leader senses that sufficient time has been allowed for that direction of flow, each person changes the position of their hands, so that their left hand is over and their right hand is under. The leader again intends aloud that the Reiki should flow, and each person lets the current flow in a clockwise direction for several minutes, or longer if you prefer.

5. You may find the current can be quite strong at times, so that the whole group can feel the need to sway counterclockwise or clockwise like a big spiralling whirlpool, so it is advisable to have your feet slightly apart to steady yourself if you are standing.

6. Because so much energy will have been generated when the whole process is complete, it is a good idea to *intend* as a group that the energy flow down each person's legs and feet into the earth, to promote healing of the planet and also to help to "ground" everyone. Finally, each person should clap their hands several times to break the connections and close down the circle. Then place your hands at midchest height in the *Gassho* (prayer) position and mentally give thanks for the Reiki, bowing slightly as a mark of respect. Afterward you should all find your Reiki energies are very high, so this would be an ideal time to carry out group or individual Reiki treatments on each other.

SHUCHU REIKI

The name *Shuchu Reiki* means:

Shuchu: concentrate/concentration, focus, center
Reiki: spiritual energy

This is a technique for giving a group treatment or concentrated Reiki to someone, often used during a Reiki course, at Reiki meetings or healing circles, and it ideally follows the *Mawashi* (see page 237), so that the group of Practitioners is channeling Reiki as effectively and strongly as possible. The idea is that two or more Practitioners work on one client, and this concentrates the Reiki energy exponentially, so that the Reiki is intensified with each additional Practitioner who joins the treatment.

1. Ideally, the client/recipient should be lying (faceup) on a massage table, made comfortable with pillows under their head and knees and a blanket to cover them, but if you don't have a massage table you can improvise appropriately.

2. Two or more Reiki Practitioners carry out a hands-on treatment, covering all the usual hand positions. The more people there are who working together, the more hand positions can be covered at the same time, so the stronger the flow of energy will be. While doing the treatment, all the Practitioners should *intend* that the Reiki flow for the highest and greatest good of the person they are working for, to encourage good health and well-being.

3. When the treatment has finished, all the Practitioners *Gassho*, give thanks for the Reiki and end with a bow of respect.

ALTERNATIVE WAYS OF USING THE HANDS WITH REIKI

The following methods can all be used during a Reiki treatment as an occasional alternative to holding your hands flat and still on or just above the body, perhaps to provide additional stimulation with Reiki on the physical body in the areas where you have found energetic disturbances when scanning. As always, while carrying out these techniques you *intend* that the Reiki will continue to flow through your hands (palms and fingertips), for the highest and greatest good of the client. Also, it is advisable to tell your client what you are intending to do, as they may not expect anything other than hands being held still, if they have had a traditional Reiki treatment before.

Another point to remember is that it would not normally be necessary or sensible to use any of these methods on physically or socially sensitive areas of the body. Naturally, there is no need for the client to remove any clothes for these techniques (or for any Reiki techniques), as the Reiki flows through clothing in the same way as when you keep your hands still.

In the *Usui Reiki Hikkei*, Dr. Usui's teaching manual, it states that Reiki emanates from all body parts, but most strongly from the hands, the eyes and the breath. You may have noticed this already. For example, I often feel Reiki flowing from my feet, as well as my hands, and my brow, heart and solar plexus chakras.

UCHI-TE CHIRYO-HO

The name *Uchi-te Chiryo-ho* means:

Uchi: strike, hit, knock, pound
Te: hand
Chiryo: medical treatment
Ho: treatment, method, way

This is a technique for patting with the hands, and it can be used for areas of numbness or where energy feels stagnant and blocked, as well as to encourage greater energy flow and movement. It can be used at any stage during a treatment, but may be best toward the end, as it will help the client to come out of a deeply relaxed state.

1. Using a firm but gentle motion (not hard enough to hurt), use the flat of the hand (palm and fingers flat) to pat and stimulate the area, starting with very soft patting and gradually getting a bit stronger, so that the motion becomes a soft slapping. Continue until you sense that it is time to move to another position (probably between 30 seconds and a minute).

2. This action stimulates both the cells of the physical body and the flow of the energy body, allowing Reiki to permeate them quickly and easily to break down blockages.

3. *Gassho*—give thanks for the Reiki and end with a bow of respect.

NADE-TE CHIRYO-HO

The name *Nade-te Chiryo-ho* means:

Nade: stroke, pat, smooth down
Te: hand
Chiryo: medical treatment
Ho: treatment, method, way

This method of stroking with the hands encourages the body's own natural energy flow, and it also promotes a greater flow of Reiki so that it quickly and easily penetrates the body. Clients often find this technique very comforting and soothing. (A reminder that there is no need for the client to remove any clothes for this, as the action is stroking rather than massage.)

1. Place your hands flat on the body. Gently, but with an acceptably firm pressure to avoid tickling, stroke your hands in a downward direction in short movements of about 5 to 10 cm (2 to 4 in), encouraging the energy flow with Reiki. Treat the client in this way either on the front or the back, from the shoulders, down the arms to the fingertips, and then from the shoulders to the waist (but *not* the breasts, if treating the front of the body on a female). Finally treat from the waist to the toes (but *not* the genital areas), giving gentle stimulation with the friction of the hands.

2. You can also use the same stroking motion from the left side to the right side, and then back again, all over the body, again making sure you don't touch any sensitive areas.

3. *Gassho*—give thanks for the Reiki and end with a bow of respect.

OSHI-TE CHIRYO-HO

The name *Oshi-te Chiryo-ho* means:

Oshi: push, pressure
Te: hand

Chiryo: medical treatment
Ho: treatment, method, way

This is a method of using slight pressure with the fingertips, pushing them gently but firmly into areas such as stiff or aching muscles or places where there is some numbness or a feeling of energy blockage or stagnation. Care must be taken not to press too hard, of course, and be aware of the necessity for reasonably short nails. This technique can also be used at any stage of a treatment, but is probably best either at the beginning or the end, so that the client is not disturbed during the more relaxing phases.

1. Place your fingertips (usually only two on each hand or on one hand only, so use either the index and middle fingers or the middle and ring fingers) or the tips of your thumbs on the area that is stiff or where you detect a blockage. Gently apply a little pressure, intending that Reiki should flow through the fingers to treat that area and/or break up energy blockages.

2. To loosen particularly stubborn stiff shoulders or aching muscles, start to gently vibrate or rotate your fingers/thumbs back and forth slightly, sending Reiki through the fingertips.

3. *Gassho*—give thanks for the Reiki, and end with a bow of respect.

ALTERNATIVE TECHNIQUES FOR USING REIKI DURING TREATMENT

KOKI-HO

The name *Koki-ho* means:

Koki: exhalation, breath, breathing
Ho: treatment, method, way

This is a method for sending healing energy with your breath, which can be particularly helpful if you are working with clients who have injuries such as burns that are painful to touch or whom you cannot touch for some other reason. You can do this technique at any time during a regular Reiki treatment, although if you are blowing into someone's face please ensure that your breath is sweet! It is also suitable for use in general "first aid" or at many other times when you wish to let Reiki flow to a person, place, object, animal, plant, etc. Note that you can add Reiki symbols to this technique—simply visualize an appropriate symbol, usually the Power Symbol, and imagine it flowing out with each breath as you silently repeat its mantra.

1. Spend a few moments breathing in through your nose and out through your mouth, pursing your lips so that they form an O shape. *Intend* that you are drawing in Reiki with every breath, and that every exhalation is filled with Reiki. When you gradually feel your chest, throat, nose and mouth become warm, you are ready to perform *Koki-ho*.

2. Continue to breathe in Reiki through your nose, and breathe gently and steadily out through your mouth, with your lips still forming an O shape, directing your breath to the area to which you wish to send Reiki.

3. Do this for one or two minutes to each area that needs this form of treatment.

4. *Gassho*—give thanks for the Reiki and end with a bow of respect.

GYOSHI-HO

The name *Gyoshi-ho* means:

Gyoshi: gaze, stare, fixation
Ho: treatment, method, way

This method for sending healing with the eyes is another one that can be used at almost any time during a Reiki treatment or for first aid or any other general purpose as well as for treating burns or injuries that cannot be touched, because it is so easy to do. Gazing with unfocused eyes is soft and gentle, and combined with love, compassion and Reiki, it can be very healing. However, it is important not to stare too hard or focus aggressively while doing *Gyoshi-ho*. A soft, gentle gaze at the area with unfocused eyes is all that is required.

1. Spend a few moments becoming centered by breathing slowly and deeply, then begin to look at the place to which you wish to send Reiki, let your eyes defocus and soften your gaze. *Intend* and feel that loving Reiki energy is pouring out through your eyes into the recipient, and "see" them perfect, whole and balanced.

2. If you have Reiki 2 (or 3) you can also visualize an appropriate symbol or symbols flowing out of your eyes into the area you are looking at, and know and *intend* that the symbol will go to the cause of the condition, for the highest and greatest good of the recipient, whatever that may be. You may notice that this technique emphasizes the loving quality of Reiki, so you feel very connected with your client.

3. Continue for one or two minutes, until you feel guided to move your gaze to the next position, or until you feel that this part of the treatment is complete.

4. *Gassho*—give thanks for the Reiki and end with a bow of respect.

TANDEN (TAN-DIEN) CHIRYO-HO

Tanden is the Japanese spelling of Tan-dien, the position just below the navel, also called the Hara or Sacral. The name *Tanden Chiryo-ho* means:

Tanden: energy vessel
Chiryo: medical treatment
Ho: treatment, method, way

This is a powerful technique for removing physical, mental or emotional poisons or toxins from both the physical and the energetic bodies. In particular, the liver and its energetic counterpart, the solar plexus chakra, can become blocked because of the ingestion of additives, preservatives, other chemicals and fumes. The brow chakra/mind can become "polluted" with negative thoughts and old patterns of behavior, and the heart chakra/heart can be blocked by negative emotions such as anger or grief. Use it for self-healing or for clients, but be warned—it often generates an urgent need to go to the toilet, and you definitely need to drink plenty of water for a day or two after this treatment! I would advise you to practice this in self-healing first so that you know how effective it can be and can discuss this with any future clients.

1. Sit or stand comfortably and spend a few moments centering yourself with your hands in the *Gassho* position, and allow your mind to become calm. Then *intend* that the Reiki should flow to remove poisons or toxins from the body for the highest and greatest good, and say silently to yourself: "I begin *Tanden Chiryo-ho* now."

2. Place one hand (it doesn't matter which) on your *Tan-dien*, 2 to 5 cm (1 to 2 in) below the navel, and the other hand on your forehead over your brow (third eye) chakra, and wait until you feel the energy beginning to build in your hands. When you feel ready, silently ask Reiki to gently flush any poisons or toxins from your physical and energy bodies, and hold this position for about five minutes, or until the energy feels balanced in both hands (sometimes it is better to hold the hands slightly away from the body).

3. Take your hand away from your forehead and put it on top of your other hand on your *Tan-dien*, and just let Reiki flow into you for as long as you feel is necessary—probably between 15 and 30 minutes.

4. *Gassho*—give thanks for the Reiki and end with a bow of respect.

HESO CHIRYO-HO

The name *Heso Chiryo-ho* means:

Heso: navel
Chiryo: medical treatment
Ho: treatment, method, way

This technique is a particularly useful one that works on what is considered in Eastern medicine to be the most important point to heal all diseases—the navel—because it is seen as the energy center of the body (that is, the location of *Tan-dien*/*Hara*/the sacral chakra). This method allows Reiki to flow directly into the *Tan-dien* to balance and harmonize the flow of Ki in the body. It requires you to sense the body's energetic pulse—the ebb and flow of Ki—which may take a bit of practice, but note that it is *not* necessary to press hard enough to feel the aortic pulse (blood flow), which can also be detected deep within the body at this point. The instructions below are for self-healing, but the process is the same for working with clients. You can place a Power Symbol into whichever hand you use, if you wish, to increase the amount of Reiki that can flow into your navel.

1. Sit or stand comfortably, and spend a few moments centering yourself with your hands in the *Gassho* position, and allow your mind to become calm. Then *intend* that the Reiki should flow into you to promote deep healing for your greatest and highest good. Say silently to yourself: "I begin *Heso Chiryo-ho* now."

2. Place one hand (usually your dominant hand) against your body, with your middle finger inserted into your navel, ensuring that you can feel your energetic pulse. (You can place your other hand elsewhere on the body, such as over your heart chakra, if you wish.) Sense that your pulse is harmonizing and balancing with Reiki, as it begins to resonate in harmony with the Universal life-force energy.

3. Hold this position until you feel relaxed and balanced, which will probably take about 5 to 10 minutes, then remove your finger from your navel.

4. *Gassho*—give thanks for the Reiki and end with a bow of respect.

NENTATSU-HO

The name *Nentatsu-ho* means:

Nen: sense, idea, thought, feeling, desire, concern, attention, care

Tatsu: discontinue, sever, cut off, abstain, interrupt, suppress, beyond
Ho: treatment, method, way

This method helps you to reprogram your thinking, and is an excellent technique for helping you to overcome bad habits, remove negativity, achieve goals, help with learning or even prevail over an illness. It works on your own (or a client's) subconscious, using Reiki with affirmations to gently reprogram the way you think, feel or react. You can repeat this exercise daily until you achieve your desired goal.

1. Decide what it is you wish to work on, and then create a positive affirmation related to that issue in the present tense, as if you have already achieved it. Some examples are: I am healthy, energized and full of vitality; I am confident and successful; I am my ideal weight and I look good and feel great; My job is fulfilling and rewarding; My life is joyful and abundant; My relationships are happy and loving.

2. Get into a comfortable position, either sitting or lying down, close your eyes and allow your breathing to become slow and steady.

3. Spend a few moments centering yourself with your hands in the *Gassho* position, allowing your mind to become calm, then say silently to yourself: "I begin *Nentatsu-ho* now."

4. Put one hand over your brow (third eye) chakra, and the other on the back of your head, at the base of the skull.

5. Then silently ask Reiki to help you to achieve what you want, based on the issue you've decided to work on. Always remember to add "for my highest and greatest good." Keep your hands in this position and repeat your affirmation(s) aloud for about five minutes, sensing the Reiki flowing into you and into your wishes and intentions.

6. Then take your hand away from your brow chakra, and place it with the other hand on the back of your head. Spend about five minutes in meditation, visualizing yourself as you will be

when you have successfully achieved your goal, or rid yourself of a bad habit. Imagine how you will feel, what you will be able to do, and so on.

7. *Gassho*—give thanks for the Reiki and end with a bow of respect.

Part V

More Steps Along the Reiki Path

Chapter 17

The Importance of
Spiritual Development

As we know, the roots of Reiki as it is practiced today began in Japan and came from a Buddhist tradition. With its lineage based in the Mystery Schools of the East, Reiki is also a spiritual discipline—a tool to encourage personal and spiritual awareness and growth, and to develop a more spiritual and meaningful way of life. But unlike most other spiritual disciplines it does not take years of study and dedication before you are granted access to it. Anyone can take Reiki, at least at First Degree level, regardless of their age, gender, nationality, spiritual background or beliefs, because Reiki is not a religion and despite its Buddhist origins it can fit into anyone's spiritual practices.

The attunement to Reiki starts a process that continues throughout life—a process of slowly raising awareness of our life purpose, of what we are here to achieve and how we can achieve it. This is working on a very subtle level and many people who don't use Reiki regularly on themselves are unaware of it. But Reiki works as a catalyst for change, bringing to the surface those aspects of life that are blocking our spiritual progress.

Sometimes this can seem a challenging process but it is always beneficial, as Reiki is Divinely guided and always works for our highest and greatest good. By this I mean that Reiki helps to bring forward in our lives what we *need*, but of course that is not necessarily always what we *want*. However, we still have a choice, as Reiki respects our right to free will.

The more you use Reiki and the more you progress by taking further training and experiencing more attunements, the more the Reiki is able to clear your energy channels and the easier it becomes for Reiki to raise your energetic vibrations to the next appropriate level. This effectively raises your consciousness, so that your connection with your Soul/Higher Self becomes closer and therefore its guidance becomes more easily accessible to you.

You may feel guided to meditate more, to explore aspects of spirituality that had not previously interested you. You may feel the need to let go of restrictions in your life that are stifling your personal and spiritual development. This might mean a real urge to change your job, see less of certain friends, take more time for yourself despite family commitments or even end a relationship that has become unhealthy or oppressive.

In addition to using Reiki, in this chapter we examine various other ways in which you can work on your personal growth and spiritual development, including meditation, visualization, and working with spirit guides and angels, but first we take a look at the tenets that Dr. Usui believed would help his students to progress spiritually—the Reiki Principles.

THE REIKI PRINCIPLES

So that their healing abilities could be increased, Dr. Usui identified a need to help his students with their personal and spiritual development, so he adopted a set of Reiki Principles from some admonishments written by the Meiji Emperor, as a guide to a sensible and suitable way of life. There are several versions of these principles in the West, but the most familiar are these two:

From the Reiki Alliance and some independent Reiki Masters:
- Just for today do not anger.
- Just for today do not worry.
- Honor your parents, teachers and elders.
- Earn your living honestly.
- Give thanks to every living thing.

From The Radiance® Technique (set up by Dr. Barbara Ray):

- Just for today I will let go of anger.
- Just for today I will let go of worry.
- Today I will count my many blessings.
- Today I will do my work honestly.
- Today I will be kind to every living creature.

The Western versions are obviously all based on what Mrs. Takata taught, but recently discovered forms in Japan, when translated, are also very similar. The following is a quote from a translation of part of Dr. Usui's memorial:

When it comes to teaching, first let the student understand well the Meiji Emperor's admonitory, then in the morning and in the evening let them chant and have in mind the five admonitions, which are:

Do not get angry today.
Do not be grievous.
Express your thanks.
Be diligent in your business.
Be kind to others.

There is also a version that comes from an original document written by Dr. Usui, which I quoted in chapter 1. You can see that there is some disparity—for example "honor your parents, teachers and elders" does not appear to be in the Japanese versions so it may have been something that Mrs. Takata instituted, but because it is so familiar to many Reiki people I have included it in the following section.

LIVING WITH THE REIKI PRINCIPLES TODAY

Although Dr. Usui asked his students to live by these principles more than 80 years ago they are as relevant to Reiki students—and others—today. Working more closely with the Reiki Principles is a valuable part of the spiritual discipline of Reiki, absorbing them into your everyday life so that they become an ordinary aspect of living. Using meditation and the Reiki symbols will help you to develop an even deeper understanding of their meanings.

Just for Today—Living in the Present

One of the most important aspects of the above principles is the phrase "Just for today"; living in the moment and being aware of what is going on around you forces you to live in the present, in the Now, which is the only time over which you have any control. Living in the present gives opportunities for appreciation and wonderment, for truly experiencing whatever you are doing at any given moment. It is a Buddhist precept—being mindful. In other words, having your mind right here, right now, not allowing your thoughts to wander into memories of time gone by or imaginings of time to come.

Just for Today Do Not Anger.

Anger is such a destructive emotion, and often we use it against those people we care about the most, so it hurts us as much as it hurts them. Anger is often generated when someone or something fails to meet our expectations—or even more important, when we do not come up to our own expectations. But anger rarely achieves anything other than to make you and others feel bad.

Anger is actually a conscious choice, a habitual response you have developed, so you have probably been reacting in a similar way to similar circumstances for years, but you can break that cycle and choose a different response instead. Then you can choose not to be angry—just for today. Use Reiki and meditation to help you to develop forgiveness and understanding of yourself and others.

Just for Today Do Not Worry.

Worry is linked with our fear of the future and the unknown, and is our usual response to a "what if" scenario—to something that might occur, but that nine times out of ten does not. Worrying is another habit we get into, yet no matter how much of it you do, the worrying itself will never achieve anything or change anything. Whatever problem or situation you are worried about—even issues such as serious health problems—if there is some action you can take to improve matters, then take it, but if there is nothing you can do about it, then there is really no other option than to "let go and let flow." Doing Reiki on yourself can help you to achieve a less anxious, more positive frame of mind.

While we continue to struggle and strive to control a situation, we are just creating an energy cycle that makes things worse— "what you resist, persists"—whereas when we let go and stop worrying about the situation, something good often comes along to sort it out. That "good" may be a person, some useful advice, a new form of treatment or just the amount of money you need. It is amazing how often just the right thing turns up. So you can choose not to worry—just for today. Use Reiki and meditation to help you discover and calm your fears, and to develop hope and trust.

Honor Your Parents, Teachers and Elders.

This does not just mean honoring older people. It really means we should honor, respect and be grateful to *everyone* for the part they play in our lives—partners, friends, neighbors, colleagues, children, shop assistants, bus drivers—in fact, every person we meet under any circumstances. All the people with whom you interact throughout your life are your teachers, whether you love them or loathe them, and every interaction is a potential learning experience because from a soul perspective all experiences, pleasant or unpleasant, contribute to the soul's growth and development.

And of course, there is a saying that "what goes around comes around," so as you honor and respect other people they will do the same for you, too. Therefore, just for today honor and respect everyone you meet and value *yourself* for the important difference *you* make to the Universe too. Use Reiki and meditation to connect with the people who have been important in your life so far, to help to heal any past hurts or misunderstandings and to permeate all your future communications.

Show Appreciation, and Count Your Blessings.

We need to value and appreciate many things in our lives and be grateful for our many blessings. However, sometimes we need to recognize those blessings first, because if life is a struggle and if we are going through a "bad patch," this colors our view of life until we assume that everything in life is bad. Even when we are happy and healthy, we are often not aware of it and take it very much for granted. Yet most of us are living very good lives, even if they are not perfect.

Take time out of every day just to stand and stare at the beauty of a flower or the happiness of a child at play. Develop an awareness of life and what it means to live it. Of course there will be ups and downs, happiness and sadness, but every experience is valuable because it helps to make you who you are. So just for today give thanks for your many blessings. The world is a wonderful place in which to live a physical life, so use Reiki and meditation to help you to develop an "attitude of gratitude," to discover and trust in the abundance of the Universe and to develop your own belief in your deservingness of love, beauty, peace and anything else you need or desire.

Earn Your Living Honestly.

Earning a living in this sense means all types of work, from paid employment and everyday tasks, like cooking a meal for ourselves or our families, to working on our self-healing with Reiki or on our self-development through meditation or reading inspirational books. We often confuse what we *do* with who we *are*, taking our sense of identity from the kind of job we have—or do not have. What we need to remember is that we are human *beings*, not human *doings*. We are *all* valuable and special; every life, every person has a role to play in the whole, and we all impact on each other in many different ways, so it is important to respect any work that we have chosen for ourselves and honor ourselves by doing our best to create a feeling of satisfaction in it.

All work is valuable to the extent that we choose to value it, so take satisfaction from even the simplest tasks, and do everything to the best of your ability. There is an old Zen Buddhist saying: "Before enlightenment chop wood, carry water; after enlightenment, chop wood, carry water." No matter how spiritual your life may become, you will still need to work in some manner to feed yourself, clothe yourself, keep yourself warm and live comfortably. Doing your work honestly also means being honest with yourself, as well as with others—it means accepting yourself for who you are. So just for today do your work honestly. Use Reiki and meditation to discover your life's purpose, so that you can *live* what you *love*.

Be Kind to Every Living Creature.

As Reiki begins to fill your life, you will start to feel more and more connected to "All That Is." As your consciousness is raised you become more aware that every living thing is a part of you, and that you are a part of it and that everything is a part of the Divine, God, the Source or whatever you choose to call it. The realization will come that there is no place for prejudice, prejudgment, cruelty or indifference in a world where we are all connected, all a part of the whole, all One. All people, animals, birds, insects and plants—and even the planet itself—have a vital role to play and should therefore be valued, respected and treated with kindness. So just for today be kind to every living creature—including yourself. Use Reiki and meditation to help you connect with all forms of living energies, and as a nurturing and loving experience for yourself.

WHAT IS MEDITATION?

Incorporating meditation into your daily routine can be a simple and effective way of enhancing your personal growth and spiritual development. Meditation is an altered state of consciousness that results in a deeply relaxed state of being that can be used to either increase or decrease your awareness of the world around you. It allows you to experience and enjoy a feeling of being at one with yourself and the Universe, and brings an acceptance of yourself and your part in "the scheme of things," leading to a deepening of "inner knowing" as opposed to simply having acquired knowledge.

Meditation is a mental and spiritual discipline that is open to anyone who is willing to try it. Successful meditation requires practice and some self-discipline, but after a while you will find it fairly easy and it becomes a natural part of daily life.

In all forms of meditation there is a focus and a quietening of the mind. This aims at first simply to reduce and eventually to eliminate the chatter of daily life and the stresses of the environment in which we live, providing a haven within which we are free to connect with our inner being. It helps us to overcome the problems and illusions we create for ourselves and that we allow others to create for us, and also helps us to overcome those habits we have formed that hold us back. Meditation allows us to go beyond the everyday into who we really are. The art of focusing and awareness of being in the moment changes brain activity, which leads to an opening of ourselves to the joy of the Universe. There are many methods of meditation, including:

- Chanting or singing using repeated simple phrases or mantras—such as chanting the Reiki symbols' mantras.

- Meditation on symbols (e.g., a cross), icons (e.g., a picture of Jesus or the Buddha) or mandalas (i.e., beautiful circular designs)—or, of course, the Reiki symbols.

- Meditation on the four elements—earth, air, fire and water (this occurs in both Eastern and Western spiritual traditions).

- Meditation with sound, such as Tibetan gongs or the sounds of nature.

- Guided meditation, usually called visualization, which takes you on a journey into your deeper self.

All methods of meditation are equally valid, so you may wish to try out a few in your search for the one that fits you the best, or you may find that a combination of forms of meditation is the way for you to develop. You can start by finding somewhere quiet and comfortable where you will not be disturbed, so you can sit or lie still for a while. It is best to have your spine straight, as this aligns the chakras and enables your *Ki* to flow properly, but it is not necessary to sit cross-legged in the lotus position. You might like to have one or two candles lit and burn some incense or relaxing essential oils. (Remember that you should never leave a burning candle or incense unattended.)

When you are ready just center yourself by beginning to breathe deeply and evenly and allow your whole body to relax. Sometimes this is best achieved by tensing your muscles first and then letting them go, starting with your feet and legs, then the trunk of your body, your shoulders and arms, and finally your neck, face and head. Allow yourself to fall into a slow, regular pattern of breathing (through your nose, not your mouth), and then begin to count each in-breath 1, 2, 3 and so on up to 9. After the ninth breath, return to 1, 2, 3 and up to 9 again, continuing like this for about five minutes.

When you are more used to meditating you can continue for much longer, but five minutes, twice a day, is a good way to start. Once you have established a habit of meditation you can try other methods, until you find one or two that you like. If you look in your local papers, there are often groups advertising meditation classes and there are plenty of books, CDs and tapes available on the subject, so if it is not something you are familiar with do give it a try.

WHAT IS VISUALIZATION?

In visualizations you either consciously and deliberately imagine something, like the visualization used in the Mental and Emotional treatment in chapter 11, or you allow your Soul/Spirit/Higher Self to influence your mind and present you with new ideas and new concepts or a different way of looking at things.

Often we will encounter a long-forgotten object or smell something that reminds us of a special time, or we will hear someone say a particular word that jogs us out of our limited realities and allows our mind to go somewhere else. We might describe this state as "daydreaming"—it is another "altered state of consciousness." Visualization is a more structured, supportive and effective vehicle for doing this, and it is easier to do than you may think.

When you begin visualizations you may have an expectation that you should "see" things very vividly, but few people do. As an exercise, close your eyes and try to remember what your bedroom looks like. Can you "see" how the furniture is arranged? Do you "know" what color the curtains are? That's visualizing!

At first you might see only part of an image or see it for only a few moments and find that the "seeing" is more a "knowing" what is there or imagining what is there, or it may be a feeling or even appear in words. All of these "sensings" are valid parts of visualization. With practice (and the more often you take yourself on visual journeys) the focus of what you "see" will become clearer, more defined and more definite.

There are many CDs and tapes available of visualizations or guided meditations, and my particular favorites are those by Gill

Edwards and Sanaya Roman, detailed in the Further Reading section (see page 305). Of course you can make your own tapes or just let your mind lead you where it wants you to go. Choose a beautiful place to imagine to start with, such as a sunlit glade in a forest or a sandy bay with the sound of gentle waves in the background, and then just "go with the flow" and enjoy it.

WORKING WITH GUIDES AND ANGELS

Some people feel called to work with angels and spirit guides (or aspects of their Soul/Spirit/Higher Self, which they choose to call guides and angels) when they do Reiki, either actually when they are using the healing energy or when they are meditating. They may even sense the presence of angels and spirit guides around them as a form of energy.

If you wish to call upon angelic beings or guides during healing, then include them in your initial intent and invocation when you start to use the Reiki, asking your angel or guide to help you with the healing work you are about to do, and remember to thank them afterward. You can also connect with a spirit guide or angel in a visualization, and there are many ways of doing this. You can ask and intend at the beginning of a visualization to meet a guide or guardian angel, and then imagine yourself meeting them in a forest glade or on top of a spiritual mountain, for example.

If you have Second Degree, you can enhance that connection by using the Reiki symbols. The following is a very powerful connection meditation I have devised, which I hope you will enjoy trying out.

Using the Symbols with Visualization

1. Make sure you are sitting or lying comfortably where you will not be disturbed for at least 20 minutes, then allow your body to relax, centering yourself by breathing deeply and evenly for a few minutes.

2. Protect yourself for your visual journey to the spiritual realms by imagining a Power Symbol in front of you and other Power Symbols behind you and on each side.

3. Draw or imagine a Distant Symbol, silently saying its mantra three times, and sending it like a bridge or rainbow up to the spiritual realms.

4. Then imagine yourself walking over that bridge, and draw or imagine a Harmony Symbol flowing across in front of you, silently saying its mantra three times to harmonize your energies with the higher vibrations of the spiritual dimension.

5. Now see or sense your guide or angel coming to meet you. You might see them as beings or as beautiful light, or just sense their loving presence.

6. Let your guide or angel lead you to a place where you can communicate with them, and ask your guide or angel to provide you with helpful insights on any problems, difficulties or questions you have at this time. Give yourself plenty of time to experience this.

7. After the communication has finished your guide or angel will lead you back to the start of your Distant Symbol bridge and may give you a sign or a gift to take back with you to the physical realms.

8. When you are about to leave thank your guide or angel for their loving help and inspiration, and turn, taking any gift or sign with you, and walk back along the Distant Symbol bridge to the place where you are sitting or lying.

9. In your imagination withdraw the Distant Symbol bridge or rainbow, and then go over in your mind what you saw or experienced, including examining and trying to interpret the significance of the sign or gift you were given.

10. Spend some time just doing Reiki on yourself, and meditate on the insights or inspiration you have received.

REINCARNATION, KARMA AND HEALING PAST LIVES

Our Soul/Spirit/Higher Self is that part of us that is directly connected to God/Goddess/All That Is. The soul is spiritual energy, and just as everything else in the Universe is energy, once that energy has been created it can only be transformed, not destroyed. Therefore the soul energy, which is the core of our being, is eternal, and it grows and develops through its experiences during each incarnation. When the physical matter, which has been its body during a single life, wears out and expires the soul moves on, eventually reincarnating into another body with which to experience physical life.

This is where the expression "past lives" comes from. Each of us alive on the planet today has probably had hundreds if not thousands of physical lives as humans, and we may have had some lives as other species too, such as animals or birds. Some people believe these can occur between episodes of human life, while others believe they were at a time before our individual soul energy started to live human lives.

There is also a belief in the East that during every incarnation each soul gathers karma, meaning that the sum of a person's actions in previous states of existence decides his or her fate in future existences. Each good thought or action is said to build up a bank of positive karma, and each bad thought or deed builds up a debt of negative karma, which then has to be worked out or repaid during many subsequent lives until that soul achieves Enlightenment.

However, in between lives, or when the soul has evolved sufficiently so that it no longer needs to experience physical life, it can still have a connection to the physical by acting as a spirit guide. This is a soul energy existing in another dimension, often referred to as the etheric or spiritual realms, whose purpose is to help humanity with guidance, inspiration, healing and so on, which is channeled through a human. However, some people believe that such spiritual guidance comes from aspects of our own infinite Soul/Higher Self that are always connected to the God-consciousness/All That Is, so that the collected wisdom of the whole Universe is always available to us, if we choose to seek it.

Past-life Healing Techniques

If you believe in reincarnation and past lives, you might like to try these two past-life healing techniques. Method A can be used after First Degree but Method B requires the use of the symbols.

Method A: Write on a piece of paper that you wish to heal any negative karma you may have collected in past lives. Hold this paper between your hands for about ten minutes and intend that Reiki should flow into those past lives for the highest and greatest good. You can repeat this exercise any number of times, until you intuitively feel that the healing has been successfully carried out.

Method B: This technique is one I have developed that can produce some very powerful healing and is probably best done in meditation:

1. Make sure you are sitting or lying comfortably where you will not be disturbed for at least 20 minutes, then allow your body to relax, centering yourself by breathing deeply and evenly for a few minutes.

2. Start by asking your spirit guides and angels to help to heal any past life (or lives) that may be producing karma for you in this life. Those angels or spirit guides who will help you with this task may appear to you in your imagination, or you may simply sense their presence.

3. Then protect yourself by imagining a Power Symbol in front of you, another behind you and one on each side.

4. Now visualize connecting to that life on a bridge made by the Distant Symbol, and send the Harmony Symbol and the Power Symbol ahead of you as you imagine yourself walking over the bridge.

5. Visualize yourself standing on the threshold of that life and, knowing that you are protected by your guides, angels and Reiki, ask to be shown in a form that is easy for you to understand any insights that might be helpful to you now in your present life. Give yourself some time to "see" those aspects of a past life (or lives) that are affecting you now.

6. Then *intend* that Reiki produce deep healing in that life (or lives), healing any karmic wounds in yourself and in any people whom you affected in that life, for the highest and greatest good.

7. Then, thanking your guides and angels for their help, turn and walk back across the Distant Symbol bridge and step off, turning back to face the bridge.

8. Send a Power Symbol across the bridge to seal in the healing, then imagine the Distant Symbol drawing back and getting smaller or fading until it disappears, so that it no longer connects you with that life.

9. Next draw a Power Symbol again in front of you to cleanse and clear the energies.

10. Finally, put one hand up in the air and bring it down forcefully, like a karate chop, to finally sever any further links with that life's karma. Heal the cut with another Power Symbol, love and light.

11. Give yourself some Reiki for about ten minutes, and don't worry if you feel very emotional, as this is quite normal. Allow those feelings to wash over you, then let them go, releasing the emotions with gratitude for the lessons they have helped you to learn.

LIFELONG HEALING

You can therefore incorporate Reiki into all aspects of your life, using it for your physical, mental, emotional and spiritual well-being. Reiki can lead you toward a deeper, more meaningful and fulfilling life. Reiki is an energy, a tool for healing, a vehicle for learning and a catalyst for change. It contains unlimited love, joy, peace, compassion, wisdom, abundance and even more. Reiki is the Divine love and light that powers the whole Universe; it is a gift of incredible power and sometimes daunting complexity, but Reiki is available to everyone when they are ready to take that next, exciting step on their spiritual journey.

Chapter 18

Becoming a Practitioner

Becoming a Reiki Practitioner can be a rewarding and interesting step to take, but if you are considering it, it is probably best to start out in a small way, integrating your practice into your life slowly, perhaps by doing treatments one or two evenings a week. That way you can start building up a regular client base and find out if you really enjoy it.

GAINING PRACTICE AND EXPERIENCE

First, though, it is sensible to get plenty of practice and experience with family and friends because any potential clients will expect you to know what you are doing, and if you feel unsure so will they. Another reason is because the more you practice the better able you will be to understand and detect subtle energies and to give each individual client what they need.

Although it is possible to become a Reiki Practitioner after Reiki 1, there are obvious advantages in waiting until you have acquired the additional skills taught at Reiki 2. I would then recommend at least six months of regular treatments on family and friends before setting up in business to take clients on a professional basis.

A realistic target to aim for in the six months would be to have carried out *at least* 30 treatments. These should be spread among a wide variety of people. Thirty treatments on one person do not actually give you any varied experience. Also, ask your friends and family to give you some honest feedback, because this information will be really valuable to ensure that you treat clients well right from the start.

What is important, however, is that you develop—and stick to—your own high standards of behavior and professional practice, ensuring that you do everything you can to treat people politely, sensitively and with great care and attention. You should also ensure that each client has as comfortable and comforting an experience as possible, so you will need to pay attention to the environment you are providing as well as to the way in which you talk to the client before and after the treatment, and the way you carry out the treatment itself.

WHERE TO SET UP YOUR PRACTICE

To start your practice in a small way it is sensible to use your own home, and it is best if you have a room you can set aside for the purpose, so that it can always be kept clean and tidy. Of course, you can set up a treatment couch in your living room but it tends not to give you such a professional feel, and if you share your living space with other people this could be tricky. You will also need to check the legal situation regarding working from home or the change of use of one of the rooms. Also, your household insurance may have to change, or there may be clauses in your home loan or rental agreements that have to be complied with.

An alternative is to take your therapy couch to clients' homes and treat them there. This does have the advantage that the client will probably feel comfortable within their own environment, but you need to check whether the space is suitable. Cramped conditions, children or dogs running around, telephones ringing or babies crying while you are trying to perform a soothing, relaxing Reiki treatment would be awful!

Another alternative is to rent a room, perhaps in a nearby complementary health clinic, but you would need plenty of clients to make this financially worthwhile. One of the most important considerations for locating your treatment room, though, is how it feels energetically. Even when they have been cleansed with Reiki, some places just don't feel right, so let yourself be guided by your intuition in this matter. If you really want to work full-time as a Practitioner, you will need to do some market research in the locality where you want to set up to find out if there is a large enough market there for you to make a worthwhile profit.

SETTING UP COSTS AND LEGAL RESPONSIBILITIES

To be a Reiki Practitioner, there are relatively few things you need, but it obviously looks more professional if you have a proper therapy couch, which can cost anywhere between £100 and £500 (in the U.S. between $250 and $750)) depending upon the type and complexity of what you buy. You will also need pillows, pillowcases, stretch-toweling sheets and one or two soft blankets, which you may already have.

You will need to be adequately insured to practice, so you must have public liability insurance, public indemnity insurance and, if you employ anyone else, employee liability insurance as well. It is good practice to have these certificates available or even discreetly displayed somewhere in your therapy room.

Insurance can usually be obtained at a reasonable cost through an umbrella organization such as the UK Reiki Federation or the Reiki Association. (Check with your initiating Master for similar organizations if you live and practice in other countries.) Another cost to bear in mind is anything you may decide to do to market your business, such as newspaper advertising or leaflets.

Don't forget that when you are in business you are legally responsible for keeping adequate financial records because you will have to calculate how much tax to pay. Accounts don't have to be difficult. A simple two-column system of income and expenditure will suffice, where you write down everything you receive on one side and all the money you have spent in running the business on the other.

Keep all your receipts and other paperwork relevant to your business, such as bank statements, check stubs, credit- and debit-card statements, invoices, gift vouchers and so on—you are legally required to keep these for seven years in the UK; you will need to check the requirements if practicing in another country.

WHAT TO CHARGE

You need to find out what other therapists charge in your area—not just for Reiki but for other therapies like reflexology and massage—because this will give you an idea about what price you can ask. This will also depend upon whether you are having to pay to rent a room, or whether you are treating people in your own home or theirs—but in the latter case, remember, it should cover your transport costs, too.

Don't fall into the trap of thinking that if you undercut all the other local therapists, you will start to attract their clients. First, that is unfair (and will probably make you unpopular in a community that might otherwise be a good support for you); second, it indicates that you don't value Reiki—or yourself—enough to charge a sensible price, and third, people may assume that as you charge less you might not be as good as the others.

Some people get very bothered by charging for Reiki treatments, but money is simply a convenient form of exchange, and if all you do is give and give and give you are putting other people under some form of obligation. Most of us have a well-developed sense of what is fair, and it can make us feel uncomfortable if we are always on the receiving end of someone's altruism.

Another side of this question is that sometimes when healing is given freely, people will take advantage of the healer, calling on his or her services constantly and expecting to be treated at almost any time, regardless of any other commitments the healer may have. Essentially, this means they have "dumped" their problems on the healer, so they don't have to take any responsibility for their own healing. This is one of the reasons why paying money for a treatment, even if it is only a small amount, actually gets them involved and builds a sense of commitment to taking part in their own healing.

Healing *is* intrinsically freely given. Reiki energy flows regardless of any financial reward. But you deserve to be paid for your time—you would be in any other job—and to be recompensed adequately for the time, effort and money you have put into training and practicing and setting up your equipment and premises. The principle is really that we should value ourselves, and learning to accept money in exchange for Reiki is a part of that valuing.

Many people find it much easier to give than to receive, so there is a meaningful lesson to learn in setting charges for Reiki treatments. The first time you ask for money can feel a bit strange, but it can be a very important step in establishing self-worth. If you still feel awkward about this, then by all means give some of your time for "free" treatments—perhaps helping out in a hospice or a nursing home for the elderly—but to be professional about your business you must set proper charges and stick to them.

MARKETING YOUR BUSINESS

To get your business off to a good start—and to keep it going—you will need to do at least a small amount of marketing, to make sure that people know where you are and what you do. There are lots of ways of bringing your services to the attention of other people.

Advertising

Placing advertisements in local newspapers or other publications is quite expensive and rarely worthwhile unless it is a specialist publication designed to publicize green issues and alternative health. Entries in directories like the Yellow Pages also cost a lot and you often have to wait at least a year before the new issue comes out. There is a growing number of opportunities to advertise in directories on the Internet, and since more and more people are using the Web this is probably a better idea. There are some addresses and sites listed in the Resources section at the back of this book.

Publicity Materials

It is certainly worth producing a good, professional leaflet—an A4 (21 × 29 cm/8½ × 11½ in) piece of paper, folded into thirds, is the most popular size. This should tell people about Reiki, about you and your background, how long treatments last and how much you charge. If you don't have much experience at producing such materials yourself, get one done by a local printing firm, because a poorly designed and produced leaflet with grammatical and spelling mistakes can really put people off.

Gift vouchers can be a good idea, so that people can buy a

treatment as a present for someone, and it is sensible to have a few letterheads (they are easy to produce on a computer) so you can send out occasional promotional letters. Business cards can be useful too because you can hand them out to groups if you give a talk, or write the next appointment time on the back before people leave.

Other Publicity

There are other ways to publicize your business, such as giving short talks to groups or taking a stand at holistic health fairs, but you need plenty of confidence for those. However, the best publicity is *always* "word of mouth"—building up a good reputation so that your clients come back for more and recommend you to other people.

Bear in mind that Reiki is not about competition—you need to trust in your potential for success, knowing that you will attract the right clients for you. The energy you put out will draw to you those people for whom you are the right person to help, so even if there is another Reiki Practitioner nearby, they will attract whoever is right for them, too. Just send Reiki to the situation and visualize nice, friendly people coming to you and that is what you will get.

GETTING YOUR TREATMENT SPACE READY

You will no doubt want to create the right atmosphere in your treatment space—an attractive blend of comfort and professionalism—so put into practice all the suggestions in chapter 7. Also, you might like to adopt the principles of feng shui, and I have suggested a few books in the Further Reading section (see page 305).

The purpose of using feng shui is to help the occupants of any building (or room) to achieve success and prosperity, so you can use the principles to create a calm, relaxing atmosphere in your therapy room. The most important principle, though, is to clear your clutter and always keep everything clean and tidy, so ensure that you clear your therapy room of all nonessential items.

WHAT DOES IT TAKE TO BE A GOOD PRACTITIONER?

If you go to a therapist of any kind, what sort of experience do you hope you will have and how do you want to be treated? Whatever your answer is, that is what it takes to be a good Practitioner. It means that you need to be a good listener, have an understanding and caring nature, be empathetic and sympathetic with people, and treat them with respect but also be knowledgeable, confident and firm enough to command their respect. And of course, you also need to be thoroughly experienced, well organized, and good at what you do.

So being experienced in the practice of Reiki is not all it takes. You also need to be competent in a wide range of other abilities, especially those that help you to deal with people, for example, coping with any emotional release, which can be one of the effects of a Reiki treatment. You may therefore wish to acquire some knowledge, experience and qualifications in related skills, such as counseling or NLP (Neuro-Linguistic Programing), to help with this side of your practice.

Another aspect of being a good Practitioner is your organizational skills. You could be a wonderfully empathetic therapist who channels Reiki beautifully, but if you are never ready when a client arrives, or worse, you are not even there because you had forgotten to write the appointment on your calendar, then you will not be seen as a good Practitioner.

THE THERAPIST-CLIENT RELATIONSHIP

Naturally, it is important to be professional at all times and that includes having set boundaries. For example, it would be unacceptable to exploit your clients either financially or emotionally by insisting on regular appointments or by making them feel dependent upon you. It is also absolutely unacceptable to interfere with or exploit a client in a sexual manner, and you should never ask a client to remove any clothing other than their coat and shoes.

Because many different types of people may come to you for treatment, it is very important that you be nonjudgmental and not show any preferences or prejudices, regardless of a person's race, color, creed, gender or sexual orientation. Your reserving judgment should also extend to accepting your clients' rights to make their own choices in regards to their health and lifestyles. Whatever opinions you might have on subjects such as smoking, heavy drinking or eating unhealthily, your clients have the right to live their lives in their own way, without being made to feel uncomfortable because of their habits.

You do have the right to ask that people not smoke or drink alcohol on your premises and to suggest that they should be sober when coming for a treatment. Of course, you also have the right to refuse to treat those whose behavior is unacceptable—for example, if they are drunk, abusive, or intimidating, or if they make you feel physically or sexually unsafe. However, it is important that you should deal with such a situation sensitively and in an uncritical way, perhaps by suggesting that another therapy or therapist might be better for the person for the time being.

CODES OF CONDUCT

As a Reiki Practitioner the most important ethical considerations are integrity, respect and confidentiality. The "status" of being a therapist puts you in a privileged position when you are treating members of the public, because you will be regarded by many as a health professional—which you are not, unless you are medically trained; whatever you say will be regarded as "the truth," so this is a considerable responsibility. Needless to say, a Practitioner must never give the impression that they have medical qualifications if they don't.

You must keep all information (medical details and appointment records) relating to each client entirely confidential, even from members of their own family, unless you have the client's consent or unless legally obliged to divulge it. A possible exception to this is if you believe there is a threat of suicide, which you are legally bound to report to an appropriate health professional such as a doctor or psychiatrist. (If you are practicing outside the UK, check to see what regulations apply in your country.)

To act with integrity you should make clear to your client what is involved in a Reiki treatment, how long it will last and how much it costs before starting a treatment, and explain what type of client records you keep. It may not be possible initially to estimate how many treatments will be needed, but it is the client's choice whether to take your advice to have further treatments or not. However, it is absolutely essential that you don't offer any diagnoses and don't claim or promise a cure.

If at any time you should feel that a client should consult a doctor, you can suggest this but do so in as calm and tactful a manner as possible. For example, if you felt a lump or unexpected mass when you placed your hands on some part of a client's body you would naturally treat the area with Reiki, but afterward you could check whether the client had detected anything there themselves. You could then calmly suggest they see a doctor to reassure themselves, saying that it is always sensible to have such things checked out.

Don't, under any circumstances, be drawn into saying what you think it might be. The best answer is always "I am sorry, I am not a doctor, so I have no idea. The best thing to do is to get it checked"—unless, of course, you are a doctor of medicine. It is not illegal for someone to refuse to get medical advice, but you must write in the client's notes that you have advised them to do so.

Another thing to remember is that clients may be nervous when coming for a treatment, so it is important to treat them with gentleness and respect, and to invite them to ask any questions or discuss anything about the treatment that may be worrying them. You will then be able to reassure them so that they can relax and enjoy the treatment.

RECORD KEEPING

All client records are confidential and should be kept where other people don't have access to them, and in the UK you are legally required to keep such records safely for seven years from the time of the last consultation (check the regulations if you live elsewhere). This also means that you should make some provision in your will for the proper disposal of your client records after your death.

Your client records—and any lists you keep of the names, addresses and telephone numbers of people who have made inquiries about treatments—are also subject to the Data Protection Act in the UK (check the situation if you practice in other countries). Even if you don't keep these lists on a computer, you may still be required to register with the Data Protection Agency.

Your initial client records should include each client's name, address, telephone number and a brief case history including any medical problems they have had in the past (and present), any surgical procedures they have undergone, any medication they are taking now and any previous medication that might be important. You should also include any alternative remedies they are taking and other complementary therapies they have received or are currently receiving. You will also need the name, address and telephone number of their doctor (for emergency use only).

Each time the client attends an appointment you should make a note of the date, time, a brief outline of the treatment and any particular results and/or experiences and any advice given. Your records should be clear and comprehensive but purely factual—no comments or opinions that even if made in a jocular way could be misinterpreted. Remember that your clients have a right to see their records if they request them, and they could also be required as part of your defense in the unfortunate (although unlikely) event of any legal action being taken against you for negligence or injury. (That, of course, is why you need public liability insurance.)

COMBINING REIKI WITH OTHER THERAPIES

Reiki works well with virtually all complementary and alternative therapies, but particularly well with any "hands-on" therapy, such as aromatherapy, reflexology, shiatsu, metamorphic technique, acupressure, craniosacral therapy, chiropractic, osteopathy and any others where massage or manipulation are involved.

If the therapist is attuned to Reiki, then the energy will automatically flow from the therapist's hands during the complementary therapy session if the client needs it. For therapies that entail taking some form of preparation internally, such as homeopathy, Bach flower remedies or herbal medicine, the bottle or container can be held in the hands to allow Reiki to flow into the medication.

If Reiki is the only therapy you practice, you might consider continuing your personal development by training in one or two others, to extend the service you can offer to your clients. I think Reiki is absolutely wonderful, but it is not the *only* thing that can help people. Sometimes an experience of a different therapy can give someone the "kick-start" they need to continue with their healing. Also, it is important to realize that all these complementary and alternative therapies have particular benefits, and to recognize and respect the contribution of other therapies, including allopathic medicine.

THE BALANCE BETWEEN REIKI AND CONVENTIONAL (ALLOPATHIC) MEDICINE

Some people seem to think that complementary and conventional medicine don't mix, but this is not the case. Many health professionals are taking an increasing interest in complementary and alternative therapies, and indeed, I have trained lots of doctors, nurses, physiotherapists and occupational therapists in Reiki. Many hospitals, hospices, clinics and doctors' surgeries now include healing and other forms of complementary therapies in their range of services on offer, and the number is growing each year.

If you do wish to carry out Reiki healing in any of these environments, however, they often require you to have qualifications in anatomy and physiology, even though a knowledge of such things is actually unnecessary for the practice of Reiki. I would suggest that it is far better to gain the extra knowledge and then put your abilities to good use, if this is something you really want to do. You will also need to carry public liability insurance, which is normal for therapists anyway.

In terms of using Reiki with someone receiving conventional medical treatment, there are some general guidelines that are important for you to follow:

- *Never* advise anyone to stop taking any medicines or to stop seeing their doctor or other health professional.

- *Never* try to diagnose what is wrong with anyone (unless you are medically qualified).

- *Always* advise clients to check with their doctor, if they wish, that receiving Reiki healing is okay, and suggest to them that when they talk to their doctor about it they refer to it as a type of spiritual healing, as many doctors will not have heard of Reiki.

- Also, *always* advise them to see a doctor if their health problem does not respond to treatment or if you intuitively feel there may be some underlying serious problem. (This must only be done in a very tactful and sensitive manner, as you don't wish to frighten them in any way and, as already indicated above, it is not your place to diagnose.)

As with complementary therapies, any prescribed medication can be held in the hands and given Reiki to enhance its beneficial effects and decrease any side effects. Simply hold it and draw the Power Symbol over it, silently saying its mantra three times and intending that Reiki should work with the medication for the highest possible good.

MEDICAL RESTRICTIONS AND NOTIFIABLE DISEASES

There are a surprising number of rules and regulations regarding what you can or cannot do as a health Practitioner, and it is essential that you get up-to-date information about any legal requirements or regulations for any country in which you wish to practice. Ignorance of the law is no defense. Your professional association should be able to help you with this, but to give you some examples, in the UK these are just some of the current instances where by treating someone with Reiki you might be going against the law:

- It is illegal to charge for the treatment of certain venereal diseases.

- Except in emergencies it is illegal to attend a woman in childbirth without qualified medical supervision.

- You cannot prescribe or sell remedies, herbs, supplements, oils, etc., unless you have appropriate qualifications.

- It is illegal to diagnose or prescribe unless medically qualified.

- Although hands-on healing of animals is permitted, an owner must have a sick animal examined by a vet, except in the case of emergencies.

- It is an offense to advertise treatments or remedies purporting cures for the following diseases: Bright's disease, cancer, cataracts, diabetes, epilepsy, glaucoma, locomotor ataxy, paralysis and tuberculosis.

- Any of the following infectious diseases must be reported to the Medical Officer of Health in your local area, and if you suspect that any client is suffering from anything on this list, you should also insist that they see a doctor: acute encephalitis, acute poliomyelitis, anthrax, cholera, diphtheria, dysentery (amoebic or bacillary), food poisoning, leprosy, leptospirosis, malaria, measles, meningitis, meningococcal septicemia (without meningitis), mumps, opthalmia neonatorum, paratyphoid fever, plague, rabies, relapsing fever, rubella, scarlet fever, smallpox, tetanus, tuberculosis, typhoid fever, typhus, viral hemorrhagic fever, viral hepatitis, whooping cough and yellow fever.

LOOKING AFTER YOURSELF

Remember the old adage "Physician, heal thyself?" Running a successful Reiki practice can be hard work, so you really need to look after yourself first—and always. You will not be much help to other people if you let yourself get run-down or become ill, so it is vital to set in motion those things that can help you to remain healthy, whole and energetic. That means concentrating on your physical well-being with good nutrition and sensible exercise, but also on your mental, emotional and spiritual well-being. You work with a wonderful holistic healing energy so please don't neglect yourself.

A daily self-treatment of a minimum of 30 to 40 minutes is important—preferably an hour, when you can—and having a regular Reiki treatment from another Practitioner is also excellent. Monthly would be fine, but if you are going through a particularly busy or stressful time try to make it once a week. Also, make sure you have a good self-cleansing routine, using the techniques recommended in chapter 15, especially before, between and after doing treatments, as this will help to keep your energies clear and balanced.

Whether you are just starting out, or have been running a busy practice for some time, one of your priorities should be to manage your time effectively to prevent burn-out. If you always find you are rushing around "chasing your tail," you need to take stock of your life and see how you can reorganize things to make your life easier.

Many of us tend to take on too much so we run ourselves ragged or begin to let other people down; the first thing to do is to start being assertive and say, "No" to everything you don't really *want* to do (and probably to some things you would like to do but simply don't have the time for). You will also need to build up your strength and stamina, as standing up doing treatments can be quite tiring otherwise. Taking up Yoga, t'ai chi, chi kung or martial arts is a good way to strengthen yourself and to get your energies flowing well.

YOUR PERSONAL SUPPORT SYSTEM

When you spend a lot of time helping others, it is essential to have your own personal support system—people you can turn to for advice and assistance if you have problems or need encouragement. Your support group should include your Reiki Master and perhaps other Practitioners or the members of a Reiki sharing group and the other students you met when you did your Reiki training, as well as family and friends. One thing that would undoubtedly help is if you could encourage some family members or friends to train in Reiki, as then you could swap treatments regularly.

YOUR FURTHER DEVELOPMENT AS A PRACTITIONER

As a Practitioner you might choose to further your development by studying other forms of Reiki, such as Karuna Reiki® (see chapter 20), or by taking courses in advanced Reiki techniques. Some Reiki Masters offer a course for Personal Mastery, sometimes called Master Practitioner, where you are taught and attuned to the Usui Master Symbol. However, you are not taught how to carry out the attunement processes, so you cannot call yourself a Reiki Master, but having the Master attunement and using the Master Symbol will enhance your capabilities. (Read the next chapter to decide whether you are ready to take on the commitment the Master attunement brings with it.) You might want to study other forms of healing or other therapies, or learn meditation or other relaxation methods, or simply read extensively about such techniques to help you improve your practice.

CONTINUING YOUR PERSONAL AND SPIRITUAL DEVELOPMENT

One of the imperatives when you start to use Reiki professionally is to work with it on your personal and spiritual development, allowing Reiki to teach you who you really are. It has the power to transform you and change your life, increasing your self-awareness and your intuition, and bringing a greater happiness and contentment. It is therefore necessary to prioritize Reiki, giving it time in your life so that you gradually develop a deeper and more meaningful relationship with it. Hopefully the last chapter will give you some ideas for your spiritual practice, plus the Japanese techniques in chapters 15 and 16.

One of the areas to be aware of is attracting clients who mirror your own problems. If you get a stream of people with the same problem, whether it be headaches, bad backs, sore throats or frozen shoulders, etc., then maybe *you* need to start looking at the metaphysical causes behind those conditions too. Perhaps you have been unwilling to look at certain areas of your life, so Reiki conveniently brings you people who can, metaphorically, push the problem under your nose so it is hard *not* to look at it.

Another area that you might give some attention to is working on your abundance issues with Reiki and visualizations: visualizing yourself attracting plenty of clients; seeing yourself as a successful Reiki Practitioner; having a good lifestyle, with a lovely home, beautiful things around you and relaxing holidays; with happy, satisfying relationships and seeing yourself fulfilling your dreams. And remember, you can use Reiki on all aspects of setting up a business, from attracting the right number of clients to attracting the appropriate funding, and even manifesting a therapy couch. (I did that and within two days someone offered me a deluxe adjustable one as an exchange for teaching them Second Degree!)

The key to much of this, as well as working on these issues with Reiki, is to feel gratitude for what you already have and to turn that feeling into something tangible. Perhaps you could tithe a proportion of the money you receive for treatments to a favorite charity or you could give some of your time to do voluntary work in hospices or nursing homes, where Reiki would be so beneficial.

Chapter 19

Third Degree Reiki

Do you *really* want to be a Reiki Master? Being a Reiki Master can be interesting, rewarding and usually great fun too, but it is not an easy path to follow and like any journey you need to be well prepared and have a good map. That is why I have put an emphasis on the word *really* in the question above, because it is not a decision to be made lightly on a whim; it definitely deserves a lot of thought.

Becoming a Reiki Master is not just about getting another, higher qualification. It is not even about being able to teach other people. It is much, much more than either of those things. Perhaps the question should read, "Do you *really* want to *commit your life* to Reiki?," because that is what it actually entails. It is a commitment for life to mastering Reiki—a commitment to a healing practice and a spiritual discipline that will inevitably change you and in all probability will change your whole life too. This is a lifetime decision, and you cannot change your mind once you have received the Master attunement.

Being a Reiki Master can be like a roller-coaster ride, and how you experience it depends very much upon your point of view. You can see it as exciting, exhilarating, enjoyable, fun, challenging and full of adventure, or you can see it as frightening and full of too many responsibilities and have an overwhelming urge to shout "I want to get off!" but of course you cannot.

Just as when you ride a roller coaster, unless you go with it, bending and turning as it does, it can be very uncomfortable; if you fight to stay upright, rigidly holding on to what you have always known, then you make the ride difficult. However, surrender to the experience, move as it moves, adapt to its speed and angles, just letting it be, and you go with the flow. That is when it becomes fun. And that is when being a Reiki Master becomes fun—when you go with the flow. That is when you are *being* a Reiki Master instead of *doing* Reiki Master. Reiki Master is not a job. It is you, *being* you. It is you *being* Reiki. It is you living what you love. And that is special. Rise to the challenge, and it can be the best kind of life you can imagine.

So if you really like the life you are living now, *don't* become a Reiki Master—at least, not yet—because change is inevitable. However, nothing stays the same forever, no matter how much we like it or dislike it. So if you love Reiki and you are curious, interested and keen enough to explore a life that is filled with Reiki—then go ahead.

THE ROLE OF A REIKI MASTER

By now you will have gathered that the role of a Reiki Master is an important one. It is a sacred responsibility for which you not only need knowledge and experience, but also wisdom, understanding, compassion and a genuine interest in people—and you need to live a life that is a good example to your students. But being a good example does *not* mean being "holier than thou" and living an ascetic life just for the sake of it.

Reiki Masters are human beings with the same foibles and failings as everyone else, so some of them smoke, some of them drink and most of them are aware that they could be looking after their bodies in better ways. But any changes they make in that direction tend to be slow and easy, and because they *want* to, not because they feel *obliged* to.

It is actually more important to show an understanding of the Reiki Principles and to use Reiki regularly, especially on yourself, than to force yourself to give up meat or caffeine-laden drinks—although that might be a direction you will be happy to follow later on in your development—because you will just end up feeling deprived. Demonstrating a balanced life, one that shows that you are trying to look after yourself and care for others, is more "real" and honest than trying to achieve some unrealistic idea of "perfection."

The role of Reiki Master is that of a respected teacher, someone who knows Reiki "inside out." By that I mean someone who lives with Reiki as an essential part of their daily lives as well as someone who has plenty of knowledge and experience of using Reiki in different ways. However, please realize that no Reiki Master knows *everything* about Reiki. Reiki is itself a teacher, so the longer a Master uses and teaches it the further along the path *toward* mastery they go.

For each Master that is a very personal journey because each comes from a different starting point. Each of us has a unique set of life experiences and it is inevitable that these will influence how, when and why we came to Reiki. Reiki Masters come from all walks of life, and this diversity means that there is bound to be a Reiki Master somewhere whose approach will appeal to you, and who will therefore be just the right person to guide you along your own personal Reiki path.

Being a Master is not just about knowing how to attune someone, or how to carry out a Reiki class. It is also about knowing how to lead people toward their own personal and spiritual fulfillment—without judgment, without censure, but with love and compassion. As a Master's self-awareness, knowledge and understanding of Reiki grow, you are even better able to carry out your role.

That is what I meant when I chose the title for this book, *Reiki for Life*. When you become attuned to Reiki you have Reiki for life; when you become a Master, Reiki gradually becomes more and more important to you, until it *is* your life.

HOW TO PREPARE FOR MASTER TRAINING

Before Reiki Master training it is especially important to raise the vibrations of your energy bodies—physical, mental, emotional and spiritual—so that you will be better prepared for the power of the Master energy coming through you. Your preparations could include daily meditation, self-treatments and practice of *Hatsurei-*

ho, plus weekly Reiki treatment "swaps" whenever possible, either with another Practitioner or preferably with the Master who will be training you. This enables you to get to know each other more, and if they have trained in the Japanese traditional techniques this would also give you the chance to receive regular *Rei-ju* attunements to increase the flow of Reiki.

In addition, you could meditate on the Reiki Principles and the Reiki Symbols, and perhaps carry out a visualization to meet your Reiki Master guides, asking them to help you with your preparation. You might also look at other possibilities for self-improvement and growth, perhaps by reading spiritually inspired books, or attending personal growth groups or workshops, plus of course thinking about the ethics, responsibilities and commitment of being a Reiki Master. Also, it would be useful to look at what experience you already have and to practice thoroughly all the techniques detailed in this book.

If you have practiced Reiki professionally for several years this would obviously be of greater benefit to your future students than if you had done only an occasional Reiki treatment on family or friends, because you would then have a wealth of experience to share with them. Equally, if you confidently and regularly use the Reiki Symbols this will enable you to teach them more effectively. I would also recommend that you get some qualifications and/or experience in teaching or training. Not only will this help your own confidence but it will also, hopefully, lead to an even better experience for your future students.

CHOOSING YOUR TYPE OF TRAINING AND INITIATING MASTER

Reiki Master training in the West can be minimal and take a very short time or very comprehensive and take a long time—or anywhere in between those two points. For example, some Masters, like me, insist that you should have at least three years' experience of Reiki, preferably as a professional Practitioner, before they will accept you for Master training, while others have no minimum time requirements and some even actively encourage every student to become a Reiki Master as soon as possible.

You therefore have several options—you can take the fast track, which could mean taking all levels of Reiki (1, 2 and 3) within a matter of a few months, weeks or even days, or you can take the slow and easy route, taking as much time as you feel you need between initiations. Whichever you choose is always at the right speed for you at a soul level, because at that level it is not possible to make mistakes—all experience is valid. However, that is not always the case at the human level, where the fast track can have some rather unpleasant consequences because your physical body has to adapt very quickly to huge changes in vibrational frequencies. This can lead to a rapid (and uncomfortable) cleansing period, not only of your physical body but also of all areas of your life. Changes are an inevitable consequence of becoming a Reiki Master—it is just the speed at which they happen that tends to be different, because in general growth needs time.

The system for Master training that was most prevalent until the early 1990s was that of Reiki Alliance Masters, who usually train by the apprenticeship system, in which a student Master works alongside a fully trained and experienced Master for at least a year, gradually learning how to organize and teach classes for Reiki 1 and 2 by observing, and then taking over certain parts of the class as they gain knowledge and confidence.

When their initiating Master considers them ready they are taught the Master Symbol and receive the Master attunement. They are also taught (and practice at Reiki classes alongside their initiating Master) the attunement processes for the first two levels. However, the attunement process for the Third Degree is often not taught until several years later, when the newly qualified Reiki Master has acquired plenty of experience.

Clearly this system limits the number of Masters who can be trained, as it would be unwieldy to have more than a couple of "trainees" working with a Master on each Reiki course, so unless they are members of the Reiki Alliance, few Masters use this type of training today. It is much more common now to learn how to be a Reiki Master in the same way as you learn the skills required in Reiki First and Second Degrees—by attending a short course. Obviously, what can be taught will be limited by the amount of time the course takes, and since this varies between one day and ten to fourteen days, with most probably taking an average of three days, there is considerable variation in content, style and quality of training.

The cost of training as a Master varies enormously, from less than £100 (U.S. $160) up to £6,000 ($10,000). However, you cannot necessarily assume that a Master who charges a high price is a good teacher offering high-quality instruction, or that one who charges a low price is an ineffective teacher offering poor instruction.

There are as many variations in Reiki Masters as there are in any other profession. There are some excellent dedicated and highly experienced Reiki teachers who charge moderate prices, whereas there are others who have little experience and offer inadequate information and poor support, yet charge high prices. I am afraid it is very much up to you to decide which is which. Probably the best way is to meditate on it and ask your Higher Self.

WHAT MIGHT BE INCLUDED IN REIKI MASTER TRAINING?

Some Masters divide the training into several parts. On the first course (usually one day) students are taught and attuned to the Usui Master Symbol, and receive instruction in a few techniques, whereafter they can call themselves "Master Practitioners." This is sometimes called Advanced Reiki Training, or ART, and usually precedes a further two-day Reiki Master training course, in which students are taught and given some time to practice the attunement processes for all three Reiki levels.

This final stage, often called "Master/Teacher," also usually includes a further two symbols—another Master Symbol with a four-syllable Japanese mantra and an Energy symbol that has a three-syllable mantra in English (although both are apparently from a Tibetan source) to which the students are attuned. Many Masters refer to this as the "Reiki Master attunement," although these symbols were never a part of the original Usui Reiki Ryoho. These short courses generally contain only very brief instructions (but no practice) on how to teach the three levels of Reiki.

Other Masters offer longer courses, some of which give you an opportunity to practice the teaching skills required. Others extend the students' knowledge to other types of Reiki (at Master level) in addition to the Usui Reiki and Tibetan Reiki referred to above, such as Tera Mai®, Sekhem, Karuna Reiki® and Jin Kei Do (all of these are described in chapter 20), including any extra symbols those systems use. There would also be some instruction in the attunement processes (normally quite different) for each system, so these are very intensive and energetically challenging courses.

There are obviously some basics that *must* be included in Reiki Master training, and other aspects that would be an advantage but that are not essential. I have put together a checklist, which you might find useful when making your decision on where to go for training:

Essential training	Possibly advantageous additions
How to draw Usui Reiki Master Symbol	How to draw Tibetan Master Symbol and Energy (Fire Serpent) Symbol
Mantra for Usui Reiki Master Symbol	Mantras for Tibetan Symbols
Attunement to the Usui Reiki Master Symbol	Attunement to the Tibetan Master Symbol and Energy (Fire Serpent) Symbol
Ways of using the Usui Master Symbol, including Master Practitioner techniques for treatments	Methods for using the Tibetan Reiki Symbols (e.g., balancing chakras, meditation)
Learning and practice of *Hui Yin* (muscular contraction to hold energy)	The single (integrated) attunement method for Usui Reiki First Degree
What to include in teaching Reiki at First Degree (individuals and classes)	The single (integrated) attunement method for Usui/Tibetan Reiki First Degree, using Tibetan Symbols
Learning and practicing the four attunement methods for Usui Reiki First Degree	The single attunement method for Usui/Tibetan Reiki Second Degree using Tibetan Symbols

Essential training	Possibly advantageous additions
What to include in teaching Reiki at Usui Reiki Second Degree (individuals and classes)	The Japanese traditional three-attunement method for Usui Reiki Second Degree
Learning and practicing the single attunement method for Usui Reiki Second Degree	Hiroshi Doi's Japanese *Rei-ju* attunement (in the Usui tradition)
The spiritual and business responsibilities of being a Reiki Master	Learning and practicing the Violet Breath
Learning and practicing the single attunement method for Usui Reiki Third Degree (does not have to be learned at same time as First and Second Degree attunement methods)	Learning the Antahkarana Symbol and its uses
What to include in teaching Reiki at Third Degree (Master) level for individuals and classes	Learning and practice of Psychic Surgery technique (removal of negative energies)
Developing the Master/Student relationship	Learning and practicing a technique called a Healing Attunement
The ongoing responsibility for personal and spiritual development	

Other opportunities may also be offered, such as observation and co-teaching of Reiki 1 and Reiki 2 courses. Something to be aware of, however, is that a significant proportion of Reiki Masters in the West don't actually use—or teach—the original Usui system for attunements, and some don't even teach the Usui Master Symbol or attune you to it. Since so many Reiki Masters have been taught the "modern" way in short courses lasting between one and three days, they use the Tibetan Reiki symbols (pioneered by William Rand), which bring through a wonderful healing energy that is somewhat "fiercer" than the very gentle, flowing Usui Reiki energy.

These symbols seem to stimulate and raise the kundalini (a very strong spiritual and sexual energy stored in the base chakra, sometimes called "serpent power"), which is wonderful, powerful and life enhancing, and can create the most profound spiritual connections. However, because it can also activate and break through the blockages in a person's sexual energy, it can occasionally have slightly unpleasant side effects on some people—mostly nausea or uncontrollable shaking for a short time. This is not entirely surprising because in the Buddhist tradition it would normally take many years of meditation and other practices to prepare for it.

THE MASTER SYMBOL

This symbol comes from the Japanese kanji, and consists of 22 strokes; it is the fourth in the Usui system of Reiki and it is described as "a Zen expression for one's own true nature or Buddha-nature of which one becomes aware during the experience of enlightenment or satori." One translation of its four-syllable mantra is "treasure house of the great beaming light."

These definitions indicate how profound this symbol is, as its use gives us direct and immediate connection to the Light, the Source, the Master within—the essence of "enlightenment." In fact, it represents that part of the self that is already completely enlightened, so when we use the Master Symbol we are actually connecting with our Higher Selves—that enlightened part of our being that has total wisdom and understanding. The Master Symbol brings in even higher and purer dimensions of light and healing—Reiki—to assist with self-awareness, personal growth, spiritual development, intuition and a deep understanding of "being," and is therefore connected with the crown chakra.

The Master Symbol can be used to bring Light into any situation. It is an essential part of all Masters' development to use this symbol to surround themselves with higher and finer vibrations as often as possible to help with self-cleansing and self-purification (on spiritual levels) in order to create a more harmonious and balanced life. Meditating on this symbol can bring enormous benefits, as it directly enters the consciousness to allow Light to enter even the darkest and most deeply buried blockages, whether those blockages are on a physical, mental, emotional or spiritual plane. It can also be used in combination with the other Reiki symbols, which will increase their effectiveness and allow them to act from only the very purest and highest motivations.

There are various ways of using the Master Symbol, once you have been attuned to it. It can be drawn in the same way as the other symbols—with the whole hand, the fingers or the eyes, or visualized. It is multidimensional energy having height, width and depth but also operating in time, space and light. It can appear to be any color, but the most usual are white, gold, purple, violet, turquoise, pink or rainbow colored.

You can draw it and "step into it," you can visualize it filling your whole being, you can imagine breathing it in with each breath, and you can draw the symbol and chant its mantra (when you are alone) to purify and fill your body and the space where you are with light, love and peace before and after any activity. It also plays a part in the attunement process for all levels of Reiki, as well as helping the Reiki Master to create a unique sacred space in which to carry out the sacred ceremony of initiation.

AFTER A REIKI MASTER COURSE

The first and most important thing to remember is that receiving a Master attunement does not make you a Reiki Master. It is just the beginning of a long journey *toward* the mastery of Reiki—a journey without end, because this amazing, Divinely guided energy is beyond mastery by humans. But we can do our best to live up to it, to "walk our talk," to "become" Reiki gradually so that it forms a vital and inexorable part of our lives.

At Master level, personal and spiritual development is no longer an option—it is a necessity. Reiki will lead you toward a more spiritual way of being through experiences that will give you a greater level of wisdom and understanding about yourself and about other people. To become a Reiki Master is to become the *embodiment* of Reiki—the embodiment of love, light, healing, harmony and balance. That might seem pretty daunting, especially at first, but at a soul level you always make the right decisions, so whenever you decide to become a Reiki Master is always the right time.

As in the cases of the other Reiki courses, after being attuned as a Reiki Master you will go through another 21-day clearing process, but it does tend to have deeper effects, as one might expect, since the Master energy has a very high vibration. I would suggest that you don't attune anyone else for a month at the very least and preferably six months or longer from the time of your attunement. Of course, you might not choose to attune anyone for many years, preferring to use the higher energies and the Master Symbol for your own personal and spiritual development and in your Reiki treatments on yourself and others, and that is fine. That is still working with the energy.

So let yourself go at a pace that suits you and don't feel pressured by family or friends, who might be looking forward to you attuning them. Only do it when you feel it is right, and trust your inner instincts, your intuition, to let you know when that is.

EXPLORING REIKI AS A SPIRITUAL DISCIPLINE

Part of a Master's personal responsibility is to explore Reiki more deeply as a spiritual discipline. The tools for this are meditation, the Reiki Principles and the four Reiki symbols and their mantras, but particularly the Master Symbol.

Because the Master Symbol works at very high and fine vibrational frequencies, it can connect you in a deep way with aspects of your Higher Self/Higher Consciousness, which usually reside in higher dimensions. This can result in a very profound personal connection to the Source/God/All That Is, leading to intense and wonderful experiences of enlightenment. These periods of illumination can last for brief seconds or for several hours, but their effects are more long lasting and, not surprisingly, can be life changing.

They can lead to amazing insights into your life path and life purpose, so that you can confidently step out on the next phase of your spiritual journey. To begin with you may need to draw the Master Symbol on a piece of paper (to be burned later) so that you can focus on it for your meditation, but after a while you will be able to visualize its image easily and to hold the image in your mind to meditate upon.

You can also chant its mantra, either silently in your mind or aloud if you are alone, which can provide a deeply relaxing meditation. You might like to try an alternative meditation technique, which is to "walk" the symbol. Imagine the Master Symbol drawn on the ground, and walk the shape of each stroke, chanting its sacred mantra as you walk. This can be done inside, but seems to be even more powerful if done outside, perhaps in a private area of a garden or in a clearing in a wood where you can be sure of being alone.

You can also meditate on the Master Symbol to entrust to Reiki any problems or difficulties you have not yet been able to solve, and the solutions will come to you intuitively. Because it connects to even higher dimensions it is especially useful for infusing any worldwide disasters with peace and healing. (The Master Symbol can eventually be used in place of the other three symbols, but it is best to leave this until much later in your development, when you have sufficient experience and practice with using all four symbols and have fully absorbed and embodied their energy.)

Other aspects of Reiki as a spiritual discipline are: daily self-treatment (preferably for at least an hour); thinking about and putting into practice the Reiki principles on a daily basis; performing at least one *Hatsurei-ho* each day, plus self-cleansing (with Reiki—and remember the cold showers too!); and using Reiki as a normal part of your everyday life so that it becomes your automatic response to anything and everything.

You can start and end each day by first placing your hands in the *Gassho* position for a few moments. Then draw (or visualize) the Master Symbol and chant its mantra with the intention that Reiki should fill your being and your day (or night). This is a really powerful way of enhancing your spiritual growth, especially if you combine it with some suitable affirmation(s) for your personal and spiritual healing, guidance and well-being.

The more you use Reiki, the more your energy channels will be cleared, opened and expanded, so that you can receive increasing amounts of energy. Eventually, you integrate Reiki into the many layers and energy fields that make up your whole self, both energetic and physical. When that happens your total being becomes Reiki, so that everything and everyone within your expanded energy field will be touched by the vibration of Reiki. You will be spreading healing, harmony and balance wherever you go. To quote Mr. Hiroshi Doi, "When everything and everyone is vibrating to its/their maximum potential, then life will cease to be a struggle, and we will experience the fullness of Who We Truly Are—Spirit having a physical experience."

Chapter 20

Other Forms of Reiki

There has been a considerable increase in interest in healing over the past 15 to 20 years, and this has been part of the reason for the spread of Reiki worldwide. However, over that period of time—and particularly since the mid-1990s—there have been many changes in, and an evolution of, the original Reiki system in the West. When in the late 1990s information finally came out of Japan, both about the real history of Dr. Usui and the healing system he started, and about techniques that we did not know, this caused great upheaval in some Reiki communities as it challenged their assumption that what they were offering was "traditional Reiki."

The situation now is probably even more confused, because "new" Reiki healing systems are being developed all the time, mostly based on the original Usui Reiki, but incorporating new symbols, different attunement methods and lots of new ideas. Add to this the claims that one system is "better" than another and counterclaims that other systems "just don't work" and it is very difficult to cut through the dross and find out what each system offers.

As I explained in an earlier chapter, because the word *Reiki* in Japanese can refer to any healing energy, most of these new healing systems are using that word to identify themselves—and also, presumably, to benefit from the reputation of the original Usui Reiki, which is well-known now in almost all countries.

I have direct experience of only a few of these new systems—I am a Karuna Reiki® Master and a Usui/Tibetan Reiki Master, as well as a Master in the original Usui Reiki Ryoho system from a Western lineage, and in the Japanese Reiki techniques through the lineage of Mr. Hiroshi Doi. However, I have tried to summarize very briefly the main points of those "offshoot" Reiki systems that exist at the time of writing this book, most of which seem to have developed in the U.S.

There are several websites that give more detail (see Resources, page 302) if you want to follow them up. I hope this will help you to identify any that you might find interesting, because there are many healing paths and one of them might be right for you. Reiki is a dynamic energy so it is bound to develop, and we will probably see even more "versions" of Reiki in the future.

Amanohuna Reiki

The word *amanohuna* means the "Abundance of the Right Way of Life." This system, which claims to have ten levels, was channeled by Arthur Cataldo in Hawaii.

Ascension Reiki

This is a new system taught in nine levels, which claims to have nine additional symbols. Its founder appears to be Jayson Suttkus, from the U.S.

Blue Star Reiki

This was originally called Blue Star Celestial Energy. It is a channeled energy supposedly originating from an Ancient Egyptian Mystery School and brought through by channeling Makuan, the spirit guide of John Williams, a Reiki Master from South Africa. This system has been modified by Gary Jirauch, who changed the name to Blue Star Reiki. It has 14 symbols (added by Gary) and two levels, both available only to Reiki Masters.

Brahma Satya Reiki

This system was channeled by Deepak Hardiker and claims to be based upon shiva-shakti (presumably linked to Hinduism), and is only taught in India and the Philippines. Little else is known about it.

Buddho-Enersense

Sometimes called EnerSense-Buddho, this system claims to be from Buddhist Lamas in Nepal, Tibet and Northern India. It was inaugurated by the Venerable Seiji Takamori, a Buddhist monk. It is a system of spiritual discipline related to healing involving meditation practice and empowerments, using ancient symbology, mantras and other aspects of Buddhist teachings and philosophy.

Golden Age Reiki

This is a system in three levels developed by Maggie Larson (who is also called Shimara) that is similar to Tera-Mai®, but with additional channeled symbols and an apparently different type of elemental energy.

Ichi Sekai Reiki

This system of four levels was started by Andrea Mikaha-Pinkham, who calls herself a Reiki Grand Master. It is based on Usui Reiki and Johrei Reiki, but with different forms of attunement and an additional Heart attunement developed by Andrea.

Jinlap Maitri Reiki

This five-level system is also known as Tibetan Reiki, and was developed by Gary Jirauch to follow on from Karuna Reiki® Mastership. It claims to be "Tibetan Reiki in the Medicine Buddha Tradition." It has 25 symbols and includes techniques such as Meridian Therapy and trauma release.

Johrei or Jo Reiki

This system seems to have been developed from a combination of Raku Kei Reiki and the Johrei religion by a man named Jim Davis in the U.S. who taught it as one level, but it was the equivalent of going from First Degree to Master in a weekend. The Johrei Fellowship does not recognize it, and it has trademarked the name Johrei so that any unauthorized usage is forbidden. It is therefore probable that this system is no longer being taught.

Karuna Reiki®

The word *karuna* means compassion, and this healing system was developed by William Lee Rand at the International Center for

Reiki Training in the U.S. It is based on two levels and nine new symbols, plus one Usui symbol and two Tibetan symbols, and the attunement system is different from that of Usui Reiki. William Rand specifies that this system should only be available to Reiki Masters, as he wishes it to be an addition to, not an alternative to, Usui Reiki. It seems to activate a different type of healing energy from that brought in by Usui Reiki—powerful and more intense than the gentle flow of Reiki—and it has an interesting spiritual dimension.

Mari-el®

This system of one degree (plus advanced techniques) and three symbols was developed by Ethel Lombardi. She was one of Mrs. Takata's original 22 Reiki Masters in the U.S., and apparently developed the system in preference to siding with either Phyllis Furumoto or Barbara Ray after Mrs. Takata's death. The name comes from Mari, meaning Mary, Mother of Christ, and El, which is said to be one of the names of God. It is not certain whether this system is still being taught.

Men Chho Reiki® or Medicine Dharma Rei Kei©

This system of three levels is supposed to be based on reconstructed teachings from Dr. Usui's notes, letters to his students and some of the rare and secret Buddhist teachings that he studied, including "The Path of the Thunderbolt of Transcendent Light that Heals the Body and Illumines the Mind." The translations have been carried out by Lama Yeshe Drugpa Thrinley Odzer, a former Shingon Buddhist priest and the Spiritual Advisor of the Men Chhos Rei Kei Institute.

New Life Reiki

This form of Reiki has four levels, and possibly as many as 150 symbols. It seems to have been started by Dr. V. Sukumaran of the International Institute of Reiki (an Indian foundation).

The Radiance Technique®, Authentic Reiki®, Real Reiki®

This form of Reiki was originated by Dr. Barbara Ray, one of Mrs. Takata's original 22 Masters in the U.S. She decided to call her system the Radiance Technique in the mid-1980s, because she described what others were teaching as "polluted"—hence, the other names, Authentic Reiki and Real Reiki. The system used to be taught at three levels, but now there are seven levels, still based on the original symbols, but with some additional ones.

Raku Kei Reiki

This system, also referred to as "The Way of the Fire Dragon," seems to have been inaugurated by Iris Ishikuro and one of her students, Cheri L. Robertson, both members of the American Reiki Master Association. Ishikuro was one of Takata's 22 original Masters and also a Johrei Fellowship Practitioner. The name *Raku* apparently means the vertical flow of energy, and *Kei* is the horizontal flow of energy in the body. It is taught at four levels, with the use of Master Frequency plates, which are supposed to switch the polarity of the body.

Reiki-Ho

This is the name given to the system of Reiki healing, also known as Iyashi No Gendai Reiki Ho, meaning the Modern Reiki Method for Healing. It was developed by Hiroshi Doi, a Reiki Master in Japan who has trained in both the Japanese and Western Reiki traditions. It is taught at four levels: Level 1 is for opening the Reiki channel; Level 2 is for enhancing the Reiki power and extending the use of Reiki; Level 3 is for reaching a higher level of vibration of consciousness and being more creative, and Level 4 is for becoming a Reiki teacher.

Reiki Jin-Kei Do©

This is an Eastern Lineage of Reiki, through Usui, Hayashi, Tekeuchi, and the Venerable Seiji Takamori to Dr. Ranga J. Premaratna, who is the present Lineage Head. The name translates as "Reiki: The Path (Integration) of Compassion and Wisdom." Its emphasis is on a spiritual way of life and progress toward enlightenment as well as healing. It has been transmitted through Buddhist Reiki Masters and therefore has a greater content of Buddhist practices.

Reiki Plus®

This is a system developed by David Jarrell, the founder of the Reiki Plus® Institute (RPI), and it is taught at four Practitioner levels and two Master levels in a total of 310 class hours, which include etheric body and soul-level healing techniques and counseling approaches. Successful Reiki students of the RPI with suitable experience are also offered the opportunity to become ministers of the Pyramids of Light Church, recognized in the U.S. as a church of natural healing founded by David Jarrell.

Saku Reiki

This is a comprehensive wellness program built around Reiki but also incorporating nutrition, exercise, herbs, crystals and other natural remedies. It was developed by Eric Bott, originally from Germany but now based in California. It is derived from Usui Reiki as well as Karuna Reiki® and Tera Mai™ and is taught at six levels over a number of years.

Satya Japanese Reiki

This is another branch of Reiki that originated in Japan, with an Eastern lineage from Usui, Eguchi, Miyazuki, Mitsui, Takahashi, Mochizuki and Sakuma. Mitsui also studied the Radiance Technique with Dr. Barbara Ray, and the teaching is similar to that. It is taught at three levels and is found mostly in India.

Seichim or Seichem or Sekhem

This system was originated by Patrick Ziegler, a student of Dr. Barbara Ray in the U.S. It is a combination of Usui Reiki and some information from Egypt with some additional symbols. It is taught at five main levels. Some of Ziegler's students have apparently made further changes.

Sun Li Chung Reiki

This is a system from Israel that has been channeled by Yosef Sharon. It is taught at five levels and claims to use thousands of symbols (for example, 1,600 symbols at Reiki 2) but the symbols are not given to the students, because they are expected to "channel" whatever they need, and undergo attunements with their spirit guides.

Tera-Mai®

This system, taught at three levels, was originated by Kathleen Ann Milner, in the U.S. It seems to be based on the Raku Kei Reiki system but with different attunement methods and more symbols, some of which are the same as those used in Karuna Reiki®. It includes energy activations to three additional strands of energy called Sakara, Angeliclight and Sophi-el.

Tibetan Reiki

This system, developed by Ralph White, claims a lineage to Tschen Li, further claiming that Tschen Li taught Dr. Usui. There are several ways of teaching this system, including one that has one level and 19 symbols and another that has 25 symbols. Although the symbols are said to be of Tibetan origin, they don't have Tibetan names. Another version of this system appears to be the same as the Usui/Tibetan Reiki developed by William Lee Rand (described below).

Usui-Do (Traditional Japanese Reiki)

This system is from the Japanese lineage (that is, not through Mrs. Takata) and has been developed by Dave King and Melissa Riggall, both of whom trained in Japan. It is a very different concept, as it has no "Masters," and it regards the attunements simply as ceremonies with the whole system being driven solely by the intent of the Practitioner, who has at his/her disposal a number of "tools" that affect the way the energy is directed. There are seven levels in a similar ranking system to that in Japanese martial arts.

Usui Shiki Ryoho (or Usui Shiki Reiki Ryoho)

This is what is usually referred to as traditional Reiki in the West, with the lineage from Usui, Hayashi and Takata to Phyllis Lei Furumoto, Mrs. Takata's granddaughter. Furumoto and another of Takata's Masters, Paul Mitchell, set up "The Office of Grand Master," which has outlined what they call the four aspects (healing practice, personal growth, spiritual discipline, and mystic order) and nine elements (oral tradition, spiritual lineage, history, principles, form of classes, money, initiation, symbols and treatment) of the Usui Reiki system, all of which they believe should be incorporated into Reiki training and practice. Masters who belong to The Reiki Alliance generally follow this system of teaching at three levels with four symbols. Some independent Reiki Masters also use this system with some minor adaptations.

Usui/Tibetan Reiki

This system, which includes two additional symbols, was developed by William Lee Rand, an American Reiki Master, and is a combination of traditional Usui Reiki, Raku Kei Reiki and his own understandings. It is taught at four levels with a different attunement system from that of Usui Reiki, although the traditional Usui system is also taught to Reiki Masters. Levels 1 and 2 are normally taught on consecutive days. Rand set up the International Center for Reiki Training, and training with Center-accredited Reiki Masters can be counted as part of the training through The National Certification Board of Therapeutic Massage and Bodywork (USA) and the American Holistic Nurses.

Vajra Reiki®

This system originally came from Johrei Reiki, and was founded, named and trademarked by Wade Ryan, who trained in India in the 1970s. He revised the Johrei Reiki system and created a "new" energy that is claimed to be particularly effective with some of the new bacteria and viruses that have appeared in recent years. It is taught at three levels and includes mantras, meditation and energy polarity.

Resources

Useful Contact Addresses and Websites

Penelope Quest, M.Sc., B.A., Cert.Ed

For information about Reiki courses, shamanic retreats and other workshops with Reiki Master Penelope Quest, and for details of all her books:

Websites: www.reiki-quest.co.uk and www.penelopequest.co.uk
E-mail: info@reik-quest.co.uk

Reiki Teachers and Practitioners

For details of other Reiki Masters and Practitioners, and useful information about Reiki and other forms of healing, you might like to try the following organizations and websites (these were all correct when going to press, but please check the websites for up-to-date information):

U.S. AND CANADA CONTACTS

Canadian Reiki Association
Box 54570, 7155 Kingsway, Burnaby, BC,
V5E 4J6
Website: www.reiki.ca
E-mail: reiki@reiki.ca

International Association of Reiki Professionals (IARP)
PO Box 481, Winchester, MA 01890
Website: www.iarp.org
E-mail: info@iarp.org

The International Center for Reiki Training (William Lee Rand)
21421 Hilltop St, #28, Southfield, MI
48034-1023

Website: www.reiki.org
E-mail: center@reiki.org

The Radiance Technique International Association Inc. (TRTIA)
PO Box 40570, St. Petersburg, FL 33743-0570
Website: www.trtia.org
E-mail: TRTIA@aol.com

The Reiki Alliance—Worldwide
PO Box 41, Cataldo,
ID 83810-1041
Website: www.reikialliance.com
E-mail: info@reikialliance.com

Reiki Center for Healing Arts
1764 Hamlet St, San Mateo, CA 94403
Website: www.reikifranbrown.com
E-mail: revfranb@pacbell.net

The Reiki Foundation
PO Box 362, Brewster, NY 10509-
0362
Website: www.asunam.com/
reiki_foundation.htm
E-mail: asunam@msn.com

Reiki Outreach International
PO Box 191156, San Diego, CA 92159-
1156
Website: www.annieo.com/reikioutreach

**Southwestern Usui Reiki Ryoho
Association**
PO Box 5162, Lake Montezuma, AZ
86342-5162
Website: www.reiho.org
E-mail: adonea@msn.com

Tera-Mai Healing Center
PMB 102-125, 9393 North 90th Street,
Scottsdale, AZ 85258
Website: www.kathleenmilner.com
E-mail: kathleenmilner@earthlink.net

Usui Shiki Ryoho (Phyllis Furumoto and
Paul Mitchell)
Website: www.usuireiki-ogm.com

Usui-Do (Traditional Japanese Reiki)
The Usui-Do Foundation, Toronto,
Ontario, Canada
Website: www.usui-do.org
E-mail: askme@usui-do.org

UK CONTACTS

**British Complementary Medicine
Association (BCMA)**
Website: www.bcma.co.uk
E-mail: chair@bcma.co.uk

Complementary Therapists Association
Website: www.complementary.assoc
.org.uk
E-mail: info@complementary.assoc.org.uk

Federation of Holistic Therapists (FHT)
Website: www.fht.org.uk
E-mail: info@fht.org.uk

**The General Regulatory Council
for Complementary Therapies
(GRCCT)**
Website: www.grcct.org
E-mail: admin@grcct.org

**Institute For Complementary
Medicine (ICM)**
Website: www.i-c-m.org.uk
E-mail: info@i-c-m.org.uk

National Federation of Spiritual Healers
Website: www.nfsh.org.uk

**The Reiki Alliance—UK
and Ireland**
Website: www.reikialliance.org.uk
E-mail: mail@reikialliance.org.uk

The Reiki Association
Website: www.reikiassociation.org.uk
E-mail: coordinator@reikiassociation
.org.uk

The Reiki Council
Website: www.reikicouncil.org.uk
E-mail: info@reikicouncil.org.uk

**Reiki Healers and Teachers Society
(RHATS)**
Website: www.reikihealers and teachers.net
E-mail: info@reikihealersandteachers
.net

The UK Reiki Federation
UK Reiki Federation, PO Box 71,
Andover, SP11 9WQ
Website: www.reikifed.co.uk
E-mail: enquiry@reikifed.co.uk

WORLDWIDE CONTACTS

Australian Reiki Connection
Website: www.australianreikiconnection
.com.au
International House of Reiki
(Frans & Bronwen Stiene)

Website: www.reiki.net.au
E-mail: info@reiki.net.au

Reiki Dharma (Frank Arjava Petter)
[Translations available in English,
Spanish and German]

Website: www.reikidharma.com
E-mail: Arjava@ReikiDharma.com

Reiki New Zealand Inc.
Website: www.reiki.org.nz
E-mail: info@reiki.org.nz

Further Reading

The following books are my recommendations from the many available on each subject. I have placed them under headings to make it easier to find the topics you want to pursue, but many of them cover several categories.

Abundance Theory, Law of Attraction and Cosmic Ordering

Boyes, Carolyn, *Cosmic Ordering in 7 Easy Steps*, Collins, 2006

Byrne, Rhonda, *The Secret*, Simon & Schuster Ltd, 2006

Cainer, Jonathan, *Cosmic Ordering*, Collins, 2006

Carlson, Richard, *Don't Sweat the Small Stuff About Money*, Hodder & Stoughton, 1998

Dyer, Dr. Wayne W. *Manifest Your Destiny*, Thorsons, 1998

Edwards, Gill, *Life Is a Gift*, Piatkus, 2007

Frank, Debbie, *Cosmic Ordering Guide to Life, Love & Happiness*, Penguin, 2007

Hicks, Esther and Jerry, *Ask and It Is Given*, Hay House, 2005

————. *The Law of Attraction*, Hay House, 2007

Horan, Paula, *Abundance Through Reiki*, Lotus Light Publications, 1995

Mohr, Barbel, *The Cosmic Ordering Service*, Hampton Road Publishing, 2001

Roman, Sanaya and Packer, Duane, *Creating Money*, H. J. Kramer, 2008

Feng Shui

Kingston, Karen, *Clear Your Clutter with Feng Shui*, Piatkus, 2008

————. *Creating Sacred Space with Feng Shui*, Piatkus, 1996

Spear, William, *Feng Shui Made Easy*, Thorsons, 1999

General Self-Help

Batmanghelidj, Dr. F., *Your Body's Many Cries for Water*, Tagman Press, 2007

Dyer, Dr. Wayne W., *Change Your Thoughts, Change Your Life*, Hay House UK Ltd, 2007

————. *You'll See It When You Believe It*, Arrow, 1990

Holford, Patrick, *New Optimum Nutrition Bible*, Piatkus 2004

McDermott, Ian and O'Connor, Joseph, *NLP and Health*, Thorsons, 2001

Healing

Angelo, Jack, *Your Healing Power*, Piatkus, 2007

Bays, Brandon, *The Journey*, Thorsons, 1999

Brennan, Barbara Ann, *Hands of Light*, Bantam Books, 1990

Chopra, Deepak, M.D., *Quantum Healing*, Bantam Books, 1990

Eden, Donna, and Feinstein, David, *Energy Medicine*, Piatkus, 2008

Gawain, Shakti, *The Four Levels of Healing*, Eden Grove Editions, 1997

Gerber, Richard M.D., *Vibrational Medicine for the 21st Century*, Piatkus, 2000

Myss, Caroline, Ph.D., *Why People Don't Heal and How They Can*, Bantam Books, 1998

Metaphysical Causes of Disease

Dethlefsen, Thorwald and Dahlke, Rudiger, M.D., *The Healing Power of Illness*, Vega Books, 2004

Hay, Louise L., *Heal Your Body*, Hay House, 1994

———. *You Can Heal Your Life*, Hay House, 2004

Shapiro, Debbie, *Your Body Speaks Your Mind*, Piatkus, 2007

Metaphysical Living

Edwards, Gill, *Living Magically*, Piatkus, 2006

———. *Stepping into the Magic*, Piatkus, 2006

Gawain, Shakti, *Living in the Light*, New World Library, 1998

Holden, Robert, *Living Wonderfully*, Thorsons, 1994

———. *Shift Happens*, Hodder & Stoughton, 2000

Jeffers, Susan, *End the Struggle and Dance With Life*, Hodder Mobius, 2005

———. *Feel the Fear . . . And Beyond*, Vermilion, 2000

———. *Feel the Fear and Do It Anyway*, Vermilion, 2007

Millman, Dan, *The Life You Were Born to Live*, H. J. Kramer, 1995

———. *No Ordinary Moments*, H. J. Kramer, 1992

Scovel-Shinn, Florence, *The Game of Life and How To Play It*, Vermilion, 2005

Reiki

Beckett, Don, *Reiki—The True Story*, Frog Books, 2009

Hall, Mari, *Reiki for Common Ailments*, Piatkus, 1999

Horan, Paula, *Empowerment through Reiki*, Lotus Light Publications, 1992

Lubeck, Walter & Petter, Frank Arjava, *Reiki Best Practices*, Lotus Press, 2003

Lubeck, Walter, Petter, Frank Arjava, and Rand, William Lee, *The Spirit of Reiki*, Pilgrims Publishing, 2004

Petter, Frank Arjava, *Reiki Fire*, Lotus Light Publications, 1997

———. *Reiki, The Legacy of Dr. Usui*, Lotus Light Publications, 1998

———. *The Original Reiki Handbook of Dr. Mikao Usui*, Lotus Press, 1999

Quest, Penelope, *Self-Healing with Reiki*, Piatkus, 2003

———. *The Basics of Reiki*, Piatkus, 2007

———. *Living the Reiki Way*, Piatkus, 2008

Steine, Bronwen and Frans, *The Reiki Sourcebook*, O Books, 2003

———. *The Japanese Art of Reiki*, O Books, 2005

Spiritual Growth

Davich, Victor N., *The Best Guide to Meditation*, Renaissance Books, 1998

Roberts, Jane, *The Nature of Personal Reality*, Amber-Allen Publishing, 1994

Roman, Sanaya, *Living with Joy*, H. J. Kramer, 1986

———. *Personal Power Through Awareness*, H. J. Kramer, 1986

———. *Soul Love*, H. J. Kramer, 1997

———. *Spiritual Growth*, H. J. Kramer, 1989

Walsch, Neale Donald, *Conversations with God—Books 1, 2 & 3*, Hodder & Stoughton, 1996, 1997, 1998

———. *Friendship with God*, Hodder & Stoughton, 1999

———. *Communion with God*, Hodder & Stoughton, 2000

———. *The New Revelations*, Hodder Mobius, 2003

Visualization and Guided Meditation

For tapes/CDs from Gill Edwards:
Website: www.livingmagically.co.uk
E-mail: LivMagic@aol.com

Address: Living Magically, Fisherbeck
  Mill, Old Lake Road, Ambleside,
  Cumbria, LA22 0DH, UK
Telephone: +44 (0)15394 31943

For tapes/CDs from Sanaya Roman and
  Duane Packer:

Website: www.orindaben.com
E-mail: staff@orindaben.com
Address: LuminEssence Productions,
  PO Box 1310, Medford, OR 97501,
  USA
Telephone: (541) 770-6700

Index